T0259418

Fatigue

Editors

MAX HIRSHKOWITZ
AMIR SHARAFKHANEH

SLEEP MEDICINE CLINICS

www.sleep.theclinics.com

Consulting Editor
TEOFILO LEE-CHIONG Jr

June 2013 • Volume 8 • Number 2

ELSEVIER

1600 John F. Kennedy Boulevard • Suite 1800 • Philadelphia, Pennsylvania, 19103-2899

http://www.theclinics.com

SLEEP MEDICINE CLINICS Volume 8, Number 2
June 2013, ISSN 1556-407X, ISBN-13: 978-1-4557-4912-6

Editor: Katie Saunders
Developmental Editor: Donald E. Mumford

Sleep Medicine Clinics (ISSN 1556-407X) is published quarterly by Elsevier Inc., 360 Park Avenue South, New York, NY 10010-1710. Months of issue are March, June, September and December. Business and Editorial Offices: 1600 John F. Kennedy Blvd., Ste. 1800, Philadelphia, PA 19103-2899. Customer Service Office: 3251 Riverport Lane, Maryland Heights, MO 63043. Periodicals postage paid at New York, NY and additional mailing offices. Subscription prices are $184.00 per year (US individuals), $91.00 (US residents), $383.00 (US institutions), $226.00 (foreign individuals), $127.00 (foreign residents), and $422.00 (foreign institutions), $226 (canadian individuals), $422 (canadian institutions), $127 (canadian residents). Foreign air speed delivery is included in all *Clinics* subscription prices. All prices are subject to change without notice. **POSTMASTER:** Send change of address to *Sleep Medicine Clinics*, Elsevier Health Sciences Division, Subscription Customer Service, 3251 Riverport Lane, Maryland Heights, MO 63043. Customer Service: **Tel: 1-800-654-2452 (U.S. and Canada); 314-447-8871 (outside U.S. and Canada). Fax: 314-447-8029. E-mail: journalscustomerservice-usa@elsevier.com (for print support); journalsonlinesupport-usa@elsevier.com (for online support).**

Reprints. For copies of 100 or more of articles in this publication, please contact the Commercial Reprints Department, Elsevier Inc., 360 Park Avenue South, New York, NY 10010-1710. Tel.: 212-633-3812; Fax: 212-462-1935; E-mail: reprints@elsevier.com.

Printed and bound by CPI Group (UK) Ltd, Croydon, CR0 4YY

Transferred to digital print 2012

PROGRAM OBJECTIVE

The goal of *Sleep Clinics of North America* is to keep practicing physicians up to date with current clinical practice by providing timely articles reviewing the state of the art in patient care.

TARGET AUDIENCE

All practicing physicians and other healthcare professionals.

LEARNING OBJECTIVES

Upon completion of this activity, participants will be able to:
1. Review psychiatric disorders and fatigue; sleep disorders and fatigue; and sleep disorders and cancer related fatigue.
2. Discuss fatigue in neurological disorders and cardio-respiratory conditions.
3. Outline universal fatigue management strategies.

ACCREDITATION

The Elsevier Office of Continuing Medical Education (EOCME) is accredited by the Accreditation Council for Continuing Medical Education (ACCME) to provide continuing medical education for physicians.

The EOCME designates this enduring material CME activity for a maximum of 15 *AMA PRA Category 1 Credit*(s)™. Physicians should claim only the credit commensurate with the extent of their participation in the activity.

All other health care professionals completing continuing education credit for this activity will be issued a certificate of participation.

DISCLOSURE OF CONFLICTS OF INTEREST

The EOCME assesses conflict of interest with its instructors, faculty, planners, and other individuals who are in a position to control the content of CME activities. All relevant conflicts of interest that are identified are thoroughly vetted by EOCME for fair balance, scientific objectivity, and patient care recommendations. EOCME is committed to providing its learners with CME activities that promote improvements or quality in healthcare and not a specific proprietary business or a commercial interest.

The planning committee, staff, authors and editors listed below have identified no financial relationships or relationships to products or devices they or their spouse/life partner have with commercial interest related to the content of this CME activity:

Farah Akhtar, MD; Diwakar D. Balachandran, MD; Lara Bashoura, MD; Sushanth Bhat, MD; Sudhansu Chokroverty, MD, FRCP; Nicole Congleton; Saadia Faiz, MD; Nilgun Giray, MD, DABSM; Katie Hartner; John Herman, MD; Charlie Lan, DO; Sandy Lavery; Hashir Majid, MD; Ellen F. Manzullo, MD; Jill McNair; Jose Melendez, MD; Sarah Nadeem, MD; Mary Rose, Psy.D; Munira Shabbir-Moosajee, MD; Mahalakshmi Narayanan; Amir Sharafkhaneh, MD, PhD; Sheila C. Tsai, MD; Surykanta Velamuri, MD.

The planning committee, staff, authors and editors listed below have identified financial relationships or relationships to products or devices they or their spouse/life partner have with commercial interest related to the content of this CME activity:

Max Hirshkowiz, PhD is on the speaker's burea of Jazz (maker of GHB).
Teofilo L. Lee-Chiong, MD is a consultant/advisor for CareCore National and Elsevier; has stock ownership in Philips Respironics; has royalties/patents in Elsevier, Wiley, Lippencott, Oxford University and CreateSpace.
Mary Rose, Psy.D has stock ownership and is on Speakers Bureau for ResMed.

UNAPPROVED/OFF-LABEL USE DISCLOSURE

The EOCME requires CME faculty to disclose to the participants:
1. When products or procedures being discussed are off-label, unlabelled, experimental, and/or investigational (not US Food and Drug Administration (FDA) approved); and
2. Any limitations on the information presented, such as data that are preliminary or that represent ongoing research, interim analyses, and/or unsupported opinions. Faculty may discuss information about pharmaceutical agents that is outside of FDA-approved labelling. This information is intended solely for CME and is not intended to promote off-label use of these medications. If you have any questions, contact the medical affairs department of the manufacturer for the most recent prescribing information.

TO ENROLL

To enroll in the Sleep Medicines Clinic Continuing Medical Education program, call customer service at 1-800-654-2452 or sign up online at http://www.theclinics.com/home/cme. The CME program is available to subscribers for an additional annual fee of USD 126.

METHOD OF PARTICIPATION

In order to claim credit, participants must complete the following:
1. Complete enrolment as indicated above.
2. Read the activity.
3. Complete the CME Test and Evaluation. Participants must achieve a score of 70% on the test. All CME Tests and Evaluations must be completed online.

CME INQUIRIES/SPECIAL NEEDS

For all CME inquiries or special needs, please contact elsevierCME@elsevier.com.

SLEEP MEDICINE CLINICS

Contributors

CONSULTING EDITOR

TEOFILO LEE-CHIONG Jr, MD
Professor of Medicine, Division of Pulmonary, Critical Care and Sleep Medicine, Department of Medicine, National Jewish Health, University of Colorado, Denver, Colorado; Chief Medical Liaison, Philips Respironics, Pennsylvania

EDITORS

MAX HIRSHKOWITZ, PhD
Director, Sleep Disorders and Research Center, Michael E. DeBakey VA Medical Center, Houston, Texas; Associate Tenured Professor, Section of Pulmonary, Critical Care, and Sleep Medicine, Baylor College of Medicine, Houston, Texas

AMIR SHARAFKHANEH, MD, PhD
Medical Director, Sleep Disorders and Research Center, Michael E. DeBakey VA Medical Center, Houston, Texas; Associate Tenured Professor, Section of Pulmonary, Critical Care, and Sleep Medicine, Baylor College of Medicine, Houston, Texas

AUTHORS

FARAH AKHTAR, MD
Pulmonary Fellow, Section of Pulmonary and Critical Care and Sleep Medicine, Baylor College of Medicine; Sleep Disorders and Research Center, Michael E. DeBakey VA Medical Center, Houston, Texas

DIWAKAR D. BALACHANDRAN, MD
Associate Professor, Department of Pulmonary Medicine, UT MD Anderson Cancer Center, Houston, Texas

LARA BASHOURA, MD
Associate Professor, Department of Pulmonary Medicine, UT MD Anderson Cancer Center, Houston, Texas

SUSHANTH BHAT, MD
NJ Neuroscience Institute at JFK Medical Center, Seton Hall University, Edison, New Jersey

SUDHANSU CHOKROVERTY, MD
NJ Neuroscience Institute at JFK Medical Center, Seton Hall University, Edison, New Jersey

SAADIA FAIZ, MD
Associate Professor, Department of Pulmonary Medicine, UT MD Anderson Cancer Center, Houston, Texas

NILGUN GIRAY, MD
Section of Pulmonary Critical Care and Sleep Medicine, Department of Medicine, Baylor College of Medicine, Houston, Texas

JOHN HERMAN, PhD
Professor of Psychiatry and Pediatrics, Board Certified in Sleep Medicine, University of Texas Southwestern Medical Center at Dallas, Dallas, Texas

MAX HIRSHKOWITZ, PhD
Director, Sleep Disorders and Research Center, Michael E. DeBakey VA Medical Center, Houston, Texas; Associate Tenured Professor, Section of Pulmonary, Critical Care, and Sleep Medicine, Baylor College of Medicine, Houston, Texas

CHARLIE LAN, DO
Assistant Professor of Medicine, Section of Pulmonary and Critical Care and Sleep Medicine, Baylor College of Medicine, Houston, Texas

TEOFILO LEE-CHIONG Jr, MD
Professor of Medicine, National Jewish Health, University of Colorado Denver School of Medicine, Denver, Colorado; Chief Medical Liaison Philips Respironics, Pennsylvania

HASHIR MAJID, MD
Assistant Professor, Department of Medicine, Aga Khan University, Karachi, Pakistan

ELLEN MANZULLO, MD
Professor, Department of General Internal Medicine, UT MD Anderson Cancer Center, Houston, Texas

JOSE MELENDEZ, MD
Sleep Medicine Fellow, Section of Pulmonary and Critical Care and Sleep Medicine, Baylor College of Medicine; Sleep Disorders and Research Center, Michael E. DeBakey VA Medical Center, Houston, Texas

SARAH NADEEM, MD
Endocrinologist, Dreyer Medical clinic, Aurora, Illinois

MARY ROSE, PsyD
Licensed Psychologist, Assistant Professor, Section of Pulmonary, Critical Care and Sleep Medicine, Department of Medicine, Baylor College of Medicine, Houston, Texas

MUNIRA SHABBIR-MOOSAJEE, MD
Assistant Professor, Department of Medicine, Aga Khan University, Karachi, Pakistan

AMIR SHARAFKHANEH, MD, PhD
Medical Director, Sleep Disorders and Research Center, Michael E. DeBakey VA Medical Center, Houston, Texas; Associate Tenured Professor, Section of Pulmonary, Critical Care, and Sleep Medicine, Baylor College of Medicine, Houston, Texas

SHEILA C. TSAI, MD
Assistant Professor of Medicine, National Jewish Health, University of Colorado Denver School of Medicine, Denver, Colorado

SURYAKANTA VELAMURI, MD
Assistant Professor of Medicine, Section of Pulmonary and Critical Care and Sleep Medicine, Baylor College of Medicine; Sleep Disorders and Research Center, Michael E. DeBakey VA Medical Center, Houston, Texas

Contents

In normal physiology, fatigue may be weakness (or weariness) from repeated exertion or a decreased response of cells, tissues, or organs after excessive stimulation or activity. Sleepiness plays a major role in nonpathological forms of mental fatigue. A thorough sleep history is an essential part of any fatigue risk-management program. Increasingly sophisticated computerized detection, monitoring, and surveillance systems provide the opportunity to help engineer new solutions to old problems.

Neurologists and primary care practitioners treating patients with neurologic diseases are often called on to address complaints of fatigue. This symptom often limits patients' independence and quality of life out of proportion to the degree of their neurologic impairment, and is a major cause of disability. Determining the cause and best treatment strategies for patients with this difficult symptom may be challenging. This review summarizes the mechanisms underlying central and peripheral fatigue, provides an overview of the nature of fatigue in common neurologic conditions, and discusses recent advances and recommendations in the treatment of fatigue affecting patients with neurologic disorders.

Because obstructive sleep apnea disrupts sleep and causes multiple awakenings, some patients with obstructive sleep apnea report insomnia. However, it also causes daytime sleepiness, and many patients describe excessive sleepiness. This model is similar to how fatigue presents in psychiatric disorders. Some patients complain of depression, mood swings, anxiety, irritability, or panic attacks and seek therapy or medications for these symptoms. However, each of these symptoms is strongly associated with fatigue. This article describes sleepiness and fatigue commonly seen in psychiatric disorders.

Fatigue is frequently reported in patients with chronic cardiorespiratory conditions. Change in muscle structure and function, deteriorated nutritional status, sleep deprivation, hypoxia (awake, exertional, and nocturnal), adverse effects of medications, and comorbid conditions are among many pathophysiologic mechanisms that may promote fatigue in patients. Comprehensive assessment of all the promoting causes is required for better understanding and management of fatigue in these patients.

Cancer-related fatigue (CRF) continues to be a major concern of patients and providers of cancer care. The symptoms are debilitating and can persist for many years after the cancer diagnosis and therapy. Further research is required to address the mechanisms of illness, including a better understanding of the complex interplay between the sleep system, circadian rhythms, inflammation, and the hypothalamic-pituitary axis. Genetic analysis and genomic studies need to be done to better understand which patients may be prone to CRF and which therapies may exacerbate these symptoms. Attention must be focused on understanding which comorbidities contribute to CRF.

Fatigue is defined by a lack of energy or a sensation of tiredness that may improve with rest. It is a prominent symptom in numerous disorders. Many individuals with cardiovascular, endocrine, psychiatric (anxiety and depression), and neurologic (multiple sclerosis) disorders experience significant, sometimes debilitating, fatigue. Fatigue can also factor prominently in some sleep disorders. A thorough sleep history, including sleep quality, sleep quantity, work schedule, and perceptions regarding sleep, is crucial for the evaluation of fatigue. Identifying and managing underlying sleep disorders may improve sleep and attenuate fatigue.

Fatigue is a highly subjective and nonspecific symptom. It can have a significant impact on an individual's quality of life. A variety of conditions can be associated with fatigue. This review focuses on fatigue related to renal disease and endocrine and hematological disorders. Special attention is paid to fatigue in the setting of chronic kidney disease, anemia, and parathyroid and other endocrine disorders. The pathophysiology of fatigue and its treatment options are described in connection with these disorders.

Fatigue (rather than sleepiness) generated in the work place may be caused primarily by overwork, related to factors such as repetitive non-novel tasks monotony, and noise sleepiness, however, is the direct result of sleep loss caused by either a loss of total sleep time or a misalignment of circadian rhythm. Type of fatigue or sleepiness is the first categorization needed before a management strategy can be designed. Inadequate total sleep time and misalignment of circadian rhythm are the most significant contributors to disastrous human error in the work place. Pharmacologic and nonpharmacologic interventions to modify fatigue and sleepiness suggest some overall improvement in alertness and performance with a variety of agents.

Fatigue is frequently reported in chronic medical conditions. Improvement of the primary condition positively affects health-related quality of life and fatigue. Interventions to achieve exercise rehabilitation robustly affect the fatigue in these patients. Improving sleep may improve the quality of life and fatigue. In some cases, medical management may use wake-promoting medications. The risks and benefits must be carefully weighed. When insomnia is contributing significantly to the overall fatigue, pharmacotherapy may be appropriate. The clinical picture is often complicated by potential interactions with other medications and contraindications. It is important for the physician to be aware of any self-medication.

Foreword

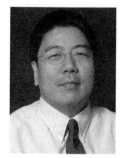

Teofilo Lee-Chiong Jr, MD
Consulting Editor

Expressions and their meanings have a tendency to linger about long after the unique circumstances that bred them have passed. These words are timeless, betraying the prejudices of the past and fossilizing the latter into the present. Truism carries many names—tired, old clichés, prosaic maxims, meaningless platitudes—even the adjectives used to characterize them have themselves become bromides. Still, they would be harmless if they were merely confined to aged textbooks. But no, these trite axioms are rediscovered in everyday speech, imparting a message that conveys the thoughtlessness of the speaker and creates insensitivity in the undiscerning listener.

Fatigue is such a term. A cursory review of its synonyms portrays a sense of desperation, helplessness, and hopelessness. A person is said to be weather-beaten, knocked up, or shattered as if fatigue were an effect alone of external forces battering the body. Other nouns reveal the opposite sense, that of an extreme self-driven activity, such as "walked off one's legs," footsore, or spent. Fatigue has been associated with sleep (drowsiness, yawning), need for breath (dyspnea, "out of breath"), cessation of work (overwork, worn out), collapse (droop, sink, swoon, faintness, syncope, ready to drop), or near-death (on one's last legs, done up). In addition to its status as a debilitating condition, fatigue has been used in other contexts, including election campaigns ("voter fatigue"), national economy ("investor fatigue"), and military campaigns ("war fatigue"). Given the wide variety of terms related to fatigue, it is easy to understand why this condition is so misunderstood by many.

"Fatigue," wrote Benjamin Franklin, "is the best pillow." Did he mean that fatigue is, in a sense, desirable since it guarantees better sleep? Other authors have provided wise counsel on how to overcome fatigue. Thomas Carlyle advised the provision of music to cure fatigue: "One is hardly sensible of fatigue while he marches to music." Or was he was referring, instead, to the curative elements of marching? Another suggested the use of tea as in Lu Yu's maxim, "Tea tempers the spirit and harmonizes the mind; dispels lassitude and relieves fatigue, awakens thought and prevents drowsiness." Flattery? Yes, it, too, was believed to relieve fatigue, according to James Monroe when he wrote, "A little flattery will support a man through great fatigue." And finally, habit, which is one of life's greatest teachers, second only to failure, has been proposed as a healing tonic. Marcus Tillius Cicero declared that, "Great is the power of habit. It teaches us to bear fatigue and to despise wounds and pain."

It is plainly apparent that we all have much to learn about fatigue, much to understand about its causes, and much to empathize with those who suffer from this medical disorder.

Teofilo Lee-Chiong Jr, MD
National Jewish Health
University of Colorado Denver
Denver, CO, USA
Philips Respironics
Pennsylvania, USA

E-mail address:
Lee-ChiongT@NJHealth.org

Sleep Med Clin 8 (2013) xi
http://dx.doi.org/10.1016/j.jsmc.2013.05.004
1556-407X/13/$ – see front matter © 2013 Published by Elsevier Inc.

Preface

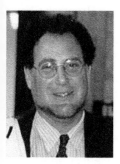
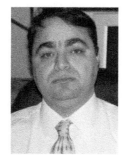

Max Hirshkowitz, PhD   Amir Sharafkhaneh, MD, PhD
Editors

In humans, sleep and fatigue represent 2 inter-twined phenomena. Although we recognize their differences, the terms are often used interchangeably. Living and working in a modern industrialized society involves engaging in many attention-intensive tasks. Some of these tasks demand sustained effort and lapses confer risk to the individual, coworkers, and/or the general public. To help mitigate such risks, fatigue risk-management procedures and occupational sleep medicine programs have evolved.

Traditionally, industrial psychologists involved in fatigue management focused on ergonomics and human factors. By contrast, sleep specialists focus on how sleep mechanisms contribute to fatigue-related performance failure. Understanding sleep homeostatic and circadian mechanisms is crucial as sleepiness is one of the most important stressors responsible for performance failure. In this volume, however, we attempt to fill the gap by discussing medical, neurologic, psychiatric, and psychological factors underlying fatigue and sleepiness. In addition, the authors review current fatigue and sleep management approaches.

We begin with an overview of fatigue and sleep definitions and concepts. I authored this article to introduce the subject fatigue management from a somewhat novel perspective and to familiarize readers with assessment methods referred to in later articles. Next, in recognition that fatigue can be a key feature in many neurologic diseases, Drs Bhat and Chokroverty, who are preeminent experts in sleep and neurologic disease (at Seton Hall University/NJ Neuroscience Institute at JFK Medical Center), review this area. Similarly, psychiatric

disorders, fatigue, and sleepiness are familiar bedfellows. Dr Herman from Southwestern Medical Center in Dallas, TX, brings his 4 decades of experience to delineate and discuss these issues. Psychiatric disorders, with their accompanying mood and/or sleep disturbances, significantly stress individuals, making them more susceptible to fatigue. Because sleep disorders, by themselves, put individuals at higher risk for fatigue-related problems, we include an article by Dr Lee-Chiong (editor of the *Sleep Review*) and his colleague at National Jewish Health, University of Colorado Denver, Dr Tsai, specifically addressing sleep disorders in relation to fatigue. Later in the volume, Drs Rose and Giray present a practical approach for psychological, cognitive, and behavioral universal fatigue and sleep management strategies.

With reference to cardiopulmonary disorders' relationship to fatigue, my colleague, Dr Sharafkhaneh, led a group to prepare a review of this association. Drs Majid, Shabbir-Moosajee, and Nadeem, from the prestigious Aga Khan University in Karachi, cover other medical disorders. My friend and colleague, Dr Balachandran, and colleagues from MD Anderson Hospital (one of the world's preeminent cancer institutes) examine our current understanding of cancer fatigue. Finally, we round out this volume by discussing medical fatigue management strategies.

It is our hope that this volume will prove useful to practitioners involved in fatigue management. We strive to include information concerning a medical approach to the issues involved. This approach attempts to augment and supplement existing paradigms for fatigue management and

Sleep Med Clin 8 (2013) xiii–xiv
http://dx.doi.org/10.1016/j.jsmc.2013.04.003
1556-407X/13/$ – see front matter © 2013 Published by Elsevier Inc.

occupational sleep medicine programs. Ultimately, we anticipate the information communicated in the volume will benefit our patients struggling against fatigue and sleepiness to live more productive and better quality lives.

Max Hirshkowitz, PhD
Director, Sleep Disorders and Research Center
Michael E. DeBakey VA Medical Center
2002 Holcombe Blvd, Building 100
Suite 6C344, Houston, Texas 77030, USA

Associate Tenured Professor
Section of Pulmonary
Critical Care, and Sleep Medicine
Baylor College of Medicine, 1 Baylor Plaza
Houston, Texas 77030, USA

Amir Sharafkhaneh, MD, PhD
Medical Director
Sleep Disorders and Research Center
Michael E. DeBakey VA Medical Center
2002 Holcombe Building, Building 100
Suite 6C344, Houston, Texas 77030, USA

Associate Tenured Professor
Section of Pulmonary
Critical Care, and Sleep Medicine
Baylor College of Medicine, 1 Baylor Plaza
Houston, Texas 77030, USA

E-mail addresses:
max.hirshkowitz@gmail.com
maxh@bcm.tmc.edu (M. Hirshkowitz)
amirs@bcm.edu (A. Sharafkhaneh)

Fatigue, Sleepiness, and Safety
Definitions, Assessment, Methodology

Max Hirshkowitz, PhD[a,b,*]

KEYWORDS

- Sleep • Fatigue • Sleep disorders

KEY POINTS

- In normal physiology, fatigue may be weakness (or weariness) from repeated exertion or a decreased response of cells, tissues, or organs after excessive stimulation, stress, or activity.
- Sleepiness plays a major role in nonpathological forms of mental fatigue.
- A thorough sleep history is an essential part of any fatigue risk-management program.
- Increasingly sophisticated computerized detection, monitoring, and surveillance systems provide the opportunity to engineer new solutions to old problems.

FATIGUE AND SLEEPINESS
Perspective

At first blush, the difference between fatigue and sleepiness seems obvious. Fatigue represents a state of tiredness, whereas sleepiness involves difficulty remaining awake. Nonetheless, institutionally we label motor vehicle mishaps resulting from drivers falling asleep as "fatigue-related accidents." When you ask a sleepy person how he or she feels, the person is likely to say "I'm tired." Similarly, when you ask a fatigued individual how he or she feels, the person is likely to say "I'm tired." Thus, in the vernacular, the terms fatigue and sleepiness are used interchangeably. The English language is rife with terms, expressions, and idioms designating fatigue, sleepiness, or both (**Table 1**). Some of these terms provide semantic nuance, other intentionally globalize for emphasis, whereas many just provide redundant variation. Such is the nature of language. However, science attempts to disambiguate to help focused analysis and quantification. Improving linguistic precision, when possible, will usually facilitate discussion.

For defining fatigue, it may help to take a page from the engineering playbook. Civil engineers and material scientists consider "fatigue" a weakening or material breakdown over time produced by repeated exposure to stressors. Thus, from one perspective, fatigue can be framed as diminished performance or increasing need for effort to maintain performance over time in response to operational environmental stressors. The critical importance of "materials fatigue" to public safety (eg, monitoring bridges, foundations, and aircraft integrity) stimulated the development of specific techniques and measurement protocols. A prime example involves measuring metal fatigue. In the laboratory, it is possible to measure structural integrity by determining changes in strength, microscopic configuration, and/or breaking point. Field measures may involve electrochemical, vibratory conduction, and spectrographic analysis. The increasing recognition of sleepiness and/or fatigue's contribution to workplace, motor vehicle, industrial, and environmental accidents has prompted development of both (1) fatigue risk-management procedures and (2) occupational sleep medicine programs.[1]

a Department of Medicine, VAMC Sleep Center 111i, 2002 Holcombe Boulevard, Houston, TX 77030, USA;
b Department of Medicine and Menninger Department of Psychiatry, Baylor College of Medicine, 1 Baylor Plaza, Houston, TX 77030, USA
* Corresponding author. VAMC– Sleep Center 111i, 2002 Holcombe Boulevard, Houston, TX 77030, USA.
E-mail address: maxh@bcm.edu

Sleep Med Clin 8 (2013) 183–189
http://dx.doi.org/10.1016/j.jsmc.2013.04.001
1556-407X/13/$ – see front matter Published by Elsevier Inc.

Table 1
Examples of some words used to describe fatigue, sleepiness, or both

Fatigued	Sleepy	Either or Both
Beat	Crashing	Exhausted
Languor	Drowsy	Burned out
Lassitude	Fading	Bushed
Lethargic	Groggy	Gassed
Listless	Narcotized	Pooped
Knackered	Heavy-headed	Played-out
Sluggish	Punchy	Tired
Weariness	Gorked	Tuckered-out
Whipped	Yawny	Wiped
Zoned	Slap happy	Zonked

This list is by no means exhaustive. The fact that many words exist and significant ambiguity in general usage suggests semantic overlap and lack of general agreement. Indeed, you (the reader) may consider some of these terms in the wrong columns.

Nonpathological Physical Fatigue

In normal physiology, fatigue may be weakness (or weariness) from repeated exertion or a decreased response of cells, tissues, or organs after excessive stimulation or activity. Furthermore, performance and/or functions recover after rest. Generally speaking, physical fatigue refers to the use of muscles to move the extremities, torso, digits, or head; however, it can involve isometric muscle contraction or reduced responsiveness at a more microscopic level. For the sake of an example, let us consider muscle fatigue. Exercise produces general muscle fatigue; continued stretching of a muscle fiber produces specific muscle fatigue. Muscle fatigue is generally understood in terms of proximal motor neuron (central) and peripheral motor unit (local) changes resulting from repeated (or intense) use that leads to diminished performance. Studies attribute the

peripheral muscle unit fatigue to muscle biochemistry, substrate depletion, lactate accumulation, electrolytic changes, acetylcholinergic synaptic alterations, and/or calcium leakage. Possible central causes are less well understood. However, it is generally agreed that exercise that exceeds conditioning or capacity more rapidly produces fatigue and will more likely provoke pain. Weight trainers frame exercise that improves conditioning as exceeding capacity mainly by increasing duration. By contrast, strength training exceeds capacity with heavier weight. Two important factors concerning fatigue that we can derive from this perspective are (1) physical fatigue often involves changes produced by exceeding capacity (if etiology is nonpathological) and (2) *sleepiness* does not necessarily induce peripheral motor unit muscle fatigue. Consequently, if we delineate physical fatigue from sleepiness one can be fatigued but not sleepy, sleepy but not fatigued, both sleepy and fatigued, or neither (**Table 2**).

Nonpathological Mental Fatigue and Sleepiness

Sleepiness plays a major role in nonpathological forms of mental fatigue. Additionally, most fatigue includes a mental component. These 2 factors likely account for why fatigue and sleepiness are so often equated. Analogous to the civil engineering definition, sleepiness acts as the stressor; however, instead of a "material breakdown" the failure lies in performance deficit. This forms the foundation for an Occupational Sleep Medicine program.

Decades ago, industrial psychologists focused on workplace design as a means of improving performance. This discipline morphed into human factors research and ultimately into what we call ergonomics. For a long time, the role of sleepiness was ignored or actively excluded because

Table 2
Factors contributing to fatigue

Behavioral Stressors	Physical and Psychological Factors	Medical and Neurologic Factors
Poor workplace design	Lack of exercise	Acute illness
Sleep deprivation	Vitamin or mineral deficiency	Anemia
Poor sleep	Boredom	Myasthenia gravis
Work volume too high	Pregnancy	Electrolyte imbalance
Work deadlines	Bereavement	Stroke
Work is high stress in nature	Depression	Poisoning
Workplace hostility	Anxiety disorder	Drug and/or medical treatments
	Relationship problems	Thyroid disease
	Personal worries	Low testosterone

reducing sleep-related performance deficit with better instrumentation design was near futile. This focus exclusively on external factors misses more than half the picture. Internal factors are ultimately more important and their interaction with external factors equally so. Bad ergonomics coupled with operator sleepiness can produce disaster. Stressful workplaces due to interpersonal issues or work intensity also increase stress and contribute to fatigue. Nonetheless, given that most ergonomic problems have been resolved, sleepiness weighs in as the chief factor in many automobile accidents, truck crashes, maritime catastrophes, aviation disasters, and health care mishaps. News headlines have made us familiar with some of these tragedies, so much so that we know them by name: Exxon Valdez oil spill, the Libby Zion case, the Three Mile Island accident, and Maggie's Law. Unfortunately, the news did not always emphasize the role of sleepiness in these incidents.[2]

Sleep Deprivation and Circadian Rhythms

Mandated Hours-of-Service rules aim to reduce sleep deprivation and thereby help decrease the potential for fatigue-related accidents. These regulatory efforts often focus particularly on those industries perceived as a risk to public safety. Thus, trucking and aviation get special scrutiny. For each truck driver killed in a crash, usually 3 or 4 other people also die. When a commercial airliner crashes, few survive. After more than 6 decades without change, the Department of Transportation's Federal Motor Carrier Safety Administration updated the Hours-of-Service Rule. Also, the Accreditation Council for Graduate Medical Education adopted an Hours-of-Service policy for resident physicians. Both of these rules clearly target sleepiness and aim to reduce sleep deprivation.

However, sleep deprivation is only half the story. The other piece of this puzzle is the circadian rhythm regulating sleepiness and alertness. Moreover, the homeostatic and circadian factors interact with respect to behavior and performance. Simply put, the homeostatic factor refers to increasing sleepiness as a function of prior wakefulness. Traditionally framed by Kleitman[3] as the "hypnotoxic theory" of sleep, the notion was that a substance builds up during wakefulness and is removed (or deactivated) by sleep. The complementary metaphor is that a substance is depleted during wakefulness and replaced during sleep. Research indicates both occur. However, during a typical day we do not become increasingly sleepy as the day progresses; that is, one is usually not sleepier at 7 PM than at noon or sleepier at noon than at 7 AM. Thus, there is another governing factor: the circadian alerting process. Under normal circumstances, the circadian alerting process begins in the morning with increasing intensity over the course of the day. This arrangement allows the circadian alerting process to offset increasing homeostatic sleep drive.[4] When this circadian alerting factor declines at night, the residual homeostatic drive is unleashed and the individual becomes very sleepy.

The circadian sleep-wake rhythm responds to light, in particular, the blue part of visual light's spectrum. Light suppresses melatonin release and melatonin suppresses the alerting action of the suprachiasmatic nucleus. Consequently, working out of synch with the circadian process can cause or exacerbate sleepiness and thereby increase the risk of performance failure. Research repeatedly demonstrates correlation between the circadian rhythm and behavioral deficits, operational errors, and accidents.

Night shift workers are at high risk.[5] Unless an individual's circadian rhythm is reversed, he or she is working without circadian assistance of alertness. In a sense, this person is a homeostatic creature and will become progressively sleepier as the work period wears on. If the person has unpaid sleep debt, the situation will be that much worse. Worse yet is if the person also has an untreated sleep disorder. To complicate matters, in the morning on returning home, the circadian alerting influence has activated. Although the person may be so sleepy that falling asleep is not an issue, several hours later problems develop. For example, after 4 to 5 hours most sleep debt may be dissipated, whereas the circadian alerting process is exerting progressively more sway. The result: insomnia. If the insomnia then produces sleep deprivation, the following night shift becomes that much more stressful. This vicious cycle sets the stage for fatigue-related performance failure. In a similar manner, other work schedules producing chaotic sleep-wake cycles also carry increased risk for fatigue-related mishaps.

General Definition and Features of Fatigue

Although fatigue has different definitions in different fields, the basic elements share common ground. Also, certain associated features provide useful perspective.

1. Fatigue is perceived as a sense of tiredness, exhaustion, or lack of energy.
2. Nonpathological fatigue improves with rest.
3. Fatigue can be provoked by exceeding capacity in terms of time-on-task or increased stress load.

4. Stress load can be increased by external factors (workplace design and work demands) and/or internal factors (medical, neurologic, and psychiatric illness; psychological stressors; and sleepiness).
5. Sleepiness is one of the most important stressors provoking fatigue.

OCCUPATIONAL SLEEP MEDICINE PROGRAMS AND FATIGUE RISK MANAGEMENT

Occupational Sleep Medicine focuses on the workplace or other operational setting. By using our understanding of sleep physiology, human factors, performance, and sleep disorders, the goals include improving health, safety, and productivity. To improve fatigue risk management, occupational medicine and sleep medicine are blended with science and outcome monitoring. Such programs would screen for relevant pathologies, develop metrics, determine risk, recommend interventions, and monitor outcomes. Much of the rest of this volume is devoted to medical, neurologic, and psychological conditions associated with fatigue and appropriate interventions. Because sleepiness often represents the most important stressor provoking fatigue, those of us involved with fatigue risk management should reflexively consider its underlying mechanisms, etiologies, and associated conditions (**Table 3**).

ASSESSMENT AND METHODS
In the Office

Sleep and work history
A thorough sleep history is an essential part of any fatigue risk-management program. The sleep history must include bedtimes and arising times (for weekdays, weekends, workdays, and nonworkdays). It is helpful to augment the sleep history with a 3-week to 4-week sleep diary; in regulatory cases, actigraphy should also be considered (see later in this article). In addition to bedtime and arising time, a sleep diary should document time taken to fall asleep; amount of time slept; number of awakenings; overall sleep quality (refreshingness); stimulant use (eg, caffeinated beverages); medication use and timing; napping; meals; work times; and exercise times, frequency, and strenuousness. The sleep diary provides an overall snapshot of the sleep-wake and work pattern. A carefully maintained diary often identifies factors negatively affecting sleep integrity and quality.

Sleep disorders screening
Administering a sleepiness questionnaire (eg, the Epworth Sleepiness Scale[6]), a fatigue questionnaire (eg, the Brief Fatigue Inventory[7]), a mood disorder instrument, an anxiety disorder screen, and some sort of generalized sleep problems questionnaire are standard procedure. Because so many workers have sleep-disordered breathing, which can cause sleepiness, administering a validated sleep apnea screening test is strongly recommended (eg, the STOP-BANG questionnaire[8]). The STOP-BANG questionnaire is particularly useful and has high sensitivity and specificity. It consists of 8 items for which 1 point is assigned for each proposition affirmed. The 8 items are as follows: (1) do you snore loudly (loud enough to be heard through closed doors); (2) are you tired, fatigued, or sleeping during the daytime; (3) has anyone observed you stop breathing in your sleep; (4) do you have or are you being treated for high blood pressure; (5) is your body mass index greater than 35 kg/m^2; (6) are you older than 50 years; (7) is your neck circumference greater than 40 cm; (8) are you male? The original article indicates that a total score above 3 indicates a high risk for sleep-related breathing disorder; however, we use a cutting score of 5 with good effect. Other paper-and-pen tests that can help detect major sleep problems include the Pittsburgh Sleep Quality Index, the International Restless Legs Scale, and the Brief Insomnia Questionnaire. These or similar psychometric tools, together with a medical history and a focused physical examination, help guide selection of subsequent diagnostic testing.

Other clinical testing
Blood, urine, and other fluids are sometimes collected to investigate possible sleep and fatigue issues. In regulatory and forensic situations, drug testing may be necessary. Clinical laboratory testing for ferritin levels when restless legs are reported, thyroid function tests for individuals

Table 3	
Causes and contributors to sleepiness	
Physiologic Causes	**Diseases and Conditions**
Insufficient sleep	Obstructive sleep apnea
Irregular sleep schedule	Narcolepsy and other hypersomnias
Environmentally disrupted sleep	Circadian rhythm disorder
Circadian mismatch	Brain injury
Stimulant withdrawal	Medical, endocrine, or infectious diseases
Sedating drug ingestion	Neurologic conditions
	Psychiatric conditions
	Severe insomnia

with fatigue, urinalysis for drug screening, and HLA typing for narcolepsy are sometimes ordered. Additionally, further medical, neurologic, and/or psychiatric testing is ordered whenever there is a clinical suspicion that such conditions or illnesses are involved.

Home Testing

Two types of home testing are relevant for occupational sleep medicine programs: actigraphy and home sleep testing (for apnea). An actigraph is a device similar to a wristwatch that records movement.[9] It can augment sleep diaries by providing objective data to confirm the self-reported diary information. Many actigraphs also monitor concurrent light-level. Thus, information about a patient's sleep schedule, rest-activity cycle, and circadian patterns can be derived from actigraphy.

Home sleep testing (for apnea) can confirm sleep-disordered breathing. Home sleep testing devices typically record airflow, respiratory effort, heart rate, snoring sounds, and oxyhemoglobin saturation. These qualify as level III devices and are sometimes called cardiopulmonary recorders. If the device also includes an electroencephalographic (EEG) channel from which wakefulness and central nervous system arousals can be scored, the device qualifies as a level II device. Level II and III devices, when used to test symptomatic individuals, provide a more economic diagnostic technique than traditional laboratory polysomnography. *However, home sleep testing cannot rule out sleep apnea because it is intrinsically less sensitive.*[10] Cardiopulmonary recorders represent the most common home apnea testing devices and these have even lower sensitivity. Nonetheless, when severe sleep apnea is present, it is readily detected (**Table 4**). We can see from the table that only a few factors can produce false-positive results, but in many circumstances sleep apnea would be mistakenly ruled out.

Chain of custody assurance constitutes a major overriding issue facing any test performed without supervision or monitoring. Because fatigue management programs can affect economics, workers, industry, and the public, legal issues can be involved. This is especially relevant in regulatory and forensic situations. The key question is... how can one be certain that data obtained from a home test device were collected from the individual to whom it was assigned? At present, to the best of our knowledge, no actigraphs and only one home sleep testing device for sleep apnea provide an adequate chain of custody apparatus.

Laboratory Sleep Testing

Polysomnography

The attended laboratory sleep study (polysomnography) is indicated for diagnosing sleep-related breathing disorders, differentiating seizures from parasomnias, and determining other disorders associated with hypersomnia.[10,11] Standard technique for recording and scoring polysomnography is summarized in the American Academy of Sleep Medicine (AASM) Scoring Manual.[12] This technique minimally includes continuous recording of brain, eye

Table 4
Situations that can produce false positive and false negative home sleep testing (for apnea) outcomes

False Positive Outcomes	False Negative Outcomes
1. Fragmented sleep can produce fall-asleep central apneas 2. Intentional breath holding 3. Without chain of custody, who was actually tested can be uncertain	1. Inadequate sleep, low SEI, long periods of wakefulness, prolonged sleep latency, and/or diminished or absent REM sleep can dilute sleep-disordered breathing index in TIB 2. Cardiopulmonary recorders do not record CNS arousals; therefore, RERA cannot be scored. 3. Subjects with good lung function and/or a brisk arousal reflex may not desaturate; consequently, hypopnea cannot be scored. 4. Subjects self-apply recording devices such that SaO2, EEG, and/or airflow problems can produce technical difficulty resulting in lower overall test sensitivity. 5. Subject can intentionally remain awake so that sleep-disordered breathing does not occur. This would not be detected with cardiopulmonary type devices. 6. Without chain of custody, who was actually tested can be uncertain

movement, breathing, cardiac, oxyhemoglobin saturation, and leg movement activity (**Table 5** for details). When possible, bedtimes and morning arising times should resemble the patient's usual habit. The patient should sleep in private, sound-attenuated, temperature-controlled bedrooms. Patients usually report to the laboratory approximately 1 hour before scheduled bedtime to complete presleep questionnaires and have monitoring devices attached by a trained technologist. Patients should maintain their usual sleep and exercise habits but abstain from alcoholic beverages, naps, and caffeinated beverages; and not have a large meal within 2 hours of testing. A presleep questionnaire provides information on adherence to these restrictions. In the morning, sensors are removed and patients complete a postsleep questionnaire concerning their impression of sleep quantity, sleep quality, and the laboratory experience.

Multiple sleep latency test and maintenance of wakefulness test

The Multiple Sleep Latency Test (MSLT) provides an objective measure for sleep tendency.[13] Clinically, it is indicated to confirm narcolepsy. The test involves 4 or 5 nap opportunities, scheduled at 2-hour intervals, commencing approximately 2 hours after the subject arises from the prior night's laboratory polysomnography. EEG, electrooculography (EOG), and electromyography (EMG)$_{submentalis}$ are recorded while the subject lies in bed and attempts to nap. Mean sleep latency of 5 minutes (or less) indicate excessive sleepiness.

The Maintenance of Wakefulness Testing (MWT) was derived from the MSLT; however, it focuses on a person's alertness in a nonstimulating situation.[13] MWT involves 4 test sessions during which a person sits in a dimly lit room and attempts to remain awake. EEG, EOG, and EMG$_{submentalis}$ are recorded during each of the 40-minute sessions (some regulatory agencies prefer 60-minute sessions) that like MSLT are scheduled at 2-hour intervals. The outcome provides objective measures of the patient's alertness and/or his or her ability to overcome drowsiness. MWT is a preferred test in regulatory situations even though successfully remaining awake on all test sessions does not guarantee safety. However, being unable to remain awake certainly raises concern and likely indicates significant risk.

MONITORING, INTERVENTION, AND THE ROAD AHEAD

Increasingly sophisticated computerized detection, monitoring, and surveillance systems provide the opportunity to engineer new solutions to old

---

Table 5
Polysomnography recording channels

Channels	Activity	Purpose
Frontal, central, and occipital EEG	Brain activity	To classify sleep stages, to recognize sleep onset, and identify CNS arousals
Left and right EOG	Eye movements	To classify sleep stages and help recognize sleep onset
Submentalis (chin) EMG	Skeletal muscle tone	To classify sleep stages and identify CNS arousals during REM sleep
Single-channel ECG	Heart rhythm	To screen for arrhythmias
Nasal-oral thermistors and nasal pressure transducer	Airflow	To identify sleep apnea, hypopnea, and respiratory effort related arousal events
Chest wall and abdominal movement and/or intercostals EMG	Respiratory effort	To differentiate central from obstructive SRBD events
Pulse oximeter (set to an averaging time of ≤ 3 s)	Oxygenation	To identify oxyhemoglobin desaturation events and score hypopnea events
Left and right anterior tibialis EMG	Leg movements	To identify activity associated with RLS and PLMD

Abbreviations: CNS, central nervous system; ECG, electrocardiography; EEG, electroencephalography; EMG, electromyography; EOG, electrooculography; PLMD, periodic limb movement disorder; REM, rapid-eye-movement; RLS, restless legs syndrome; SRBD, sleep-related breathing disorder.

problems. Advances in miniaturization, network communication, wireless connectivity, and satellite technology provide critical mass for creating a safer tomorrow. Massive computing power is available by "cloud" interface. What is needed now is defining biomarkers, risk quotients, and operational situation predictors that reliably foretell danger so that appropriate intervention can occur. We are already seeing this in motor vehicles that can monitor driver performance. Whether it is accomplished by steering parameters, surveillance of eye closure, head nodding, or by electrophysiological means, some systems have already launched to the commercial market. Of course, eliminating the driver altogether may be the ultimate solution for eliminating fatigue-related motor vehicle accidents.

But for now, fatigue-related errors, accidents, and disasters remain a part of our world. However close or far we may be from a technological solution, what we need most is a change in our attitudes and behaviors concerning sleep. Until the culture values sleep and recognizes its importance to all activities of daily living, carnage on the highways, explosions at industrial sites, mistakes in the emergency room, and aviation accidents will continue to happen.

REFERENCES

1. Belenky G, Akerstedt T. Occupational sleep medicine: introduction. In: Kryger MH, Roth T, Dement WC, editors. Principles and practice of sleep medicine. 5th edition. St Louis (MO): Elsevier Saunders; 2011. p. 734–7.

2. Walsh JK, Dement WC, Dinges DF. Sleep medicine, public policy, and public health. In: Kryger MH, Roth T, Dement WC, editors. Principles and practice of sleep medicine. 5th edition. St Louis (MO): Elsevier Saunders; 2011. p. 716–24.

3. Kleitman N. Sleep and wakefulness. Chicago: University of Chicago Press; 1939.

4. Czeisler CA, Buxton OM. The human circadian timing system and sleep-wake regulation. In: Kryger MH, Roth T, Dement WC, editors. Principles and practice of sleep medicine. 5th edition. St Louis (MO): Elsevier Saunders; 2011. p. 402–19.

5. American Academy of Sleep Medicine. International classification of sleep disorders, 2nd edition: diagnostic and coding manual. Westchester (IL): American Academy of Sleep Medicine; 2005.

6. Johns MW. A new method for measuring daytime sleepiness: the Epworth Sleepiness Scale. Sleep 1991;14:540–5.

7. Mendoza T, Wang XS, Cleeland CS, et al. The rapid assessment of fatigue severity in cancer patients: use of the Brief Fatigue Inventory. Cancer 1999;85: 1186–96.

8. Chung F, Yegneswaran B, Liao P, et al. STOP questionnaire: a tool to screen obstructive sleep apnea. Anesthesiology 2008;108:812–21.

9. Hirshkowitz M. Introduction to sleep medicine diagnostics in adults. In: Barkoukis TJ, Matheson JK, Ferber R, et al, editors. Therapy in sleep medicine. Philadelphia: Elsevier; 2012. p. 28–40.

10. Hirshkowitz M, Sharafkhaneh A. Comparison of portable monitoring with laboratory polysomnography for diagnosing sleep-related breathing disorders: scoring and interpretation. Sleep Med Clin 2011;6:283–92.

11. Standards of Practice Committee of the American Academy of Sleep Medicine. Practice parameters for the indications for polysomnography and related procedures: an update for 2005. Sleep 2005;28: 499–521.

12. Iber C, Ancoli-Israel S, Chesson A, et al. The AASM manual for the scoring of sleep and associated events: rules, terminology and technical specifications. 1st edition. Westchester (IL): American Academy of Sleep Medicine; 2007.

13. Hirshkowitz M, Sarwar A, Sharafkhaneh A. Evaluating sleepiness. In: Kryger MH, Roth T, Dement WC, editors. Principles and practice of sleep medicine. 5th edition. St Louis (MO): Elsevier Saunders; 2011. p. 1624–31.

Fatigue in Neurologic Disorders

Sushanth Bhat, MD*, Sudhansu Chokroverty, MD

KEYWORDS

- Neurologic fatigue • Central fatigue • Peripheral fatigue • Chronic fatigue syndrome
- Neuroimaging in fatigue • Fatigue in multiple sclerosis • Fatigue and basal ganglia
- Postpolio fatigue

KEY POINTS

- Fatigue is a common complaint and a major source of morbidity in patients with neurological disorders. It is independent of neurologic disability and is often very limiting, with a significant impact on quality of life.
- It is crucial that health care providers regularly enquire into the presence and adequate treatment of fatigue in their patients with neurologic disorders.
- Fatigue must be distinguished from weakness, muscle fatigability, depression and excessive daytime sleepiness, all of which may coexist in neurologic disease.
- In most neurologic disorders, both central and peripheral fatigue play a role.
- Treatment of the underlying neurologic disease and fatigue must proceed in a complementary manner.
- Several pharmacological agents have been tried to treat fatigue in a variety of disorders, but for most patients with central fatigue, a combination of cognitive behavioral therapy and a graded exercise program seem to be most efficacious.

INTRODUCTION

Chronic fatigue is a common complaint reported by patients seen in primary care and neurology practices. Although various studies have indicated that it is present in 21% to 38% of primary care patients,[1,2] with up to 18% complaining of fatigue lasting greater than 6 months,[2] measurement of the prevalence of this symptom is made difficult by the lack of a standard definition, both among patients and the medical community. The term fatigue may be used by patients to describe muscle weakness, inability to sustain voluntary activity (muscle fatigability), exercise intolerance, excessive daytime sleepiness, inability to concentrate and perceived cognitive deficits, apathy, lack of energy or a loss of motivation, all of which may be the result of a variety of neurologic and medical disorders. In many cases, the underlying disorder is already known and being treated; in such cases, optimization of ongoing treatment may be the best approach. However, more perplexing for physicians is when complaints of fatigue seem to be without immediate discernable cause; this has led to a tendency to consider the symptom a manifestation of somatization, leading to frustration on the part of both the patient and the practitioner. On the flip side, many patients with chronic fatigue do not report it to their physicians; studies indicate that this figure may be as high as 52% in certain cancer populations, with only 14% receiving specific advice about, or treatment of this symptom.[3] Optimal treatment strategies for chronic fatigue are controversial and still evolving, as is our understanding of the nature and underlying mechanisms responsible for this disabling symptom.

Disclosures: None.
NJ Neuroscience Institute at JFK Medical Center, Seton Hall University, 65 James Street, Edison, NJ 08818, USA
* Corresponding author.
E-mail address: sbhat2012@yahoo.com

NEUROLOGIC DEFINITIONS OF FATIGUE

Defining fatigue is important when dealing with neurologic disease. In dealing with fatigue as a symptom, it is helpful to classify it as peripheral or central in nature. Another distinction that is often made is between physical and mental fatigue, with the latter being an exclusive feature of central fatigue.[4] These terms are described in greater detail in the following sections of this review article.

Peripheral Fatigue

At the most basic level, peripheral fatigue is attributable to a failure of a component of the motor unit (Fig. 1). The anterior horn cell is the final common pathway for voluntary activity. Nerve impulses in the form of action potentials travel along motor axons in peripheral nerves and end at neuromuscular junctions, where the postsynaptic muscle membrane is depolarized chemically by the presynaptic release of acetylcholine, which binds with its receptors on the muscle. Multiple individual miniature end plate potentials result, which summate to produce a full end plate potential in the postsynaptic membrane and culminate in an all-or-none action potential, if the threshold potential is crossed. Muscle then contracts through interlocking of actin and myosin filaments aided by the release of calcium into the sarcoplasm. This is an active process requiring adenosine triphosphate expenditure. Common sites of peripheral fatigue are abnormal action potential initiation and transmission in the anterior horn cell and motor axon, failure of the neuromuscular junction, and metabolic changes in the muscle, leading to defects in excitation-contraction coupling.

The recording and comparison of force generated by electrical stimulation of muscle before and after exercise is the principal manner of detecting peripheral fatigue. Typically, after a pre-exercise electrical stimulation, the individual performs a maximum voluntary contraction (MVC) for a predetermined period, usually 30 or 60 seconds, which is measured with a force transducer. A subsequent

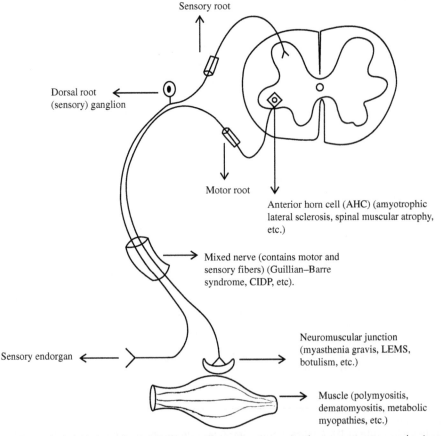

Fig. 1. The motor unit (consisting of anterior horn cell, motor root, mixed nerve, neuromuscular junction, and muscle) with common causes of fatigue listed at each site. CIDP, chronic inflammatory demyelinating neuropathy; LEMS, Lambert-Eaton myasthenic syndrome. See text for detailed description. (*Modified from* Chaudhuri A, Behan PO. Fatigue in neurological disorders. Lancet 2004;363(9413):978–88; with permission.)

postexercise electrical stimulation is then performed, and the force generated is compared with the pre-exercise tracing. Lower amplitudes of the waveform and slow relaxation phases are characteristic of peripheral fatigue (**Fig. 2**).[5]

Central Fatigue

Central fatigue can be thought of as arising from the central nervous system (CNS) (ie, the motor systems proximal to the anterior horn cells). It implicates the brain and spinal cord. A key concept in understanding central fatigue is that of central activation failure (CAF), which is increased during exercise or sustained muscle activity in central fatigue. With CAF, there is suboptimal CNS output to the motor unit, resulting in muscle fatigue.

CAF can be measured by analyzing the force generated during MVC and providing superimposed electrical stimulation (tetanic fusion at 50 Hz for 500 milliseconds). The resulting twitch interpolation is then analyzed; the absence of a significant twitch amplitude suggests full voluntary contraction and no central fatigue, whereas a large superimposed twitch suggests significant CAF (see **Fig. 2**). One well-designed study showed that in normal individuals who were asked to perform a 4-minute isometric MVC of the tibialis anterior muscle, approximately 20% of the decrease in MVC-generated force after exercise was attributable to central causes (measured by a twitch interpolation technique), and the rest was determined to be peripheral fatigue caused by metabolic changes

within the muscle itself, mainly changes in intracellular pH. There was no failure of transmission across the neuromuscular junction, as shown by lack of decrease in compound muscle action potential (CMAP) amplitudes.[6] Even in normal individuals, both central and peripheral causes contribute to muscle fatigability, although the contributions of each remain to be clearly defined. Patients with CNS disorders like multiple sclerosis (MS), Parkinson disease (PD), and possibly chronic fatigue syndrome (CFS) experience physical fatigue that may not be explainable by neurologic deficits. Although the mechanisms underlying central fatigue remain unclear, cortical stimulation techniques have been used to study their role ("SEE SECTION ON CORTICAL STIMULATION STUDIES IN FATIGUE").

THE SITES OF FATIGUE

The finer pathophysiologic details underlying fatigue are likely to vary in each disease state. Nevertheless, recent research has shed some light into the basic mechanisms likely to be contributing to neurologic fatigue.[3] Fatigue seems to be the result of diffuse as well as multifocal dysfunction across large neuroanatomic pathways, as well as dysregulation in both neurologic and endocrinologic feedback systems, with immunologic abnormalities playing a role in certain disease processes.[7]

Voluntary activity is the result of a fine interplay between various central and peripheral neurologic loci. Physical activity is the ultimate output of this system, which is dependent on feedback control

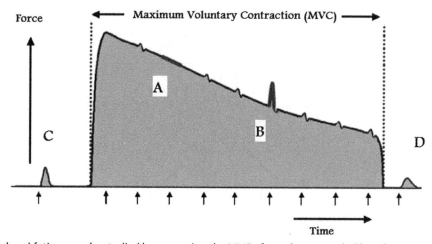

Fig. 2. Peripheral fatigue can be studied by measuring the MVC of muscle as recorded by a force transducer. Note the normal linear decrease in force generated attributable to peripheral fatigue. Superimposed tetanic stimulation (*arrows*) is used to detect the presence of central fatigue. Absence of significant twitch amplitude (A) suggests the absence of central activation failure (CAF), whereas a large twitch amplitude (B) suggests the presence of CAF. A pre-MVC tetanic contraction (C) and post-MVC tetanic contraction (D) are compared. The lower amplitude and slower relaxation phase of the post-MVC contraction is suggestive of the development of peripheral fatigue. (*Modified from* Zwarts MJ, Bleijenberg G, van Engelen BG. Clinical neurophysiology of fatigue. Clin Neurophysiol 2008;119:2–10; with permission.)

from several areas, including cognitive input. Although the primary motor cortex is the initiator of voluntary activity, cognitive influences and internal motivation are required to convert an intended action into a physical movement. These influences may be pathologically altered in psychiatric disorders or with certain centrally active medications, contributing to the overall perception of fatigue. **Fig. 3** denotes the major areas of dysfunction at the central level that may contribute to fatigue. As is evident, influences from the limbic areas, the prefrontal cortex, the hypothalamus, the brainstem, and the cerebellum all exert their influences on motor output and, when lesioned, may decrease motivational drive and contribute to fatigue. In addition to influencing motivation and internal drive through mechanisms yet to be fully understood, these areas are intricately involved with the generation and fine-tuning of voluntary movement, and neurologic examination of the patient in clinic helps distinguish focal deficits (causing weakness and imbalance) from fatigue. Pyramidal weakness (with hyperreflexia and spasticity, as well as preferential weakness in the extensors of the arm and flexors of the leg) is seen with lesions of the motor cortex and its descending pathways, whereas hypotonia and dyscoordination are seen in cerebellar diseases. Basal gangliar lesions cause a variety of extrapyramidal findings, including tremors, rigidity, and abnormal movements (chorea, hemiballismus, and athetosis). Yet fatigue is often seen in neurologic disease even in the absence of these findings,

suggesting a mechanism independent of motor dysfunction. The basal ganglia, in particular, have become the focus of recent interest, based on their central role in higher-order, cognitive control of motor function.[4] Areas subserving arousal and attention (ie, ascending reticular activating system and the limbic system) are particular areas of focus inasmuch as their dysfunction is naturally expected to limit motivation and cognitive drive to work.[8]

In addition, afferent input from peripheral receptors (sensory end organs, including the retina, cochlea, cutaneous receptors, and muscle spindles) regulates the continuous smooth flow of impulses along the neural pathways required to maintain physical activity. An imbalance of any of these inputs, either at the receptor level or the pathways leading to central processing (including the spinal cord, brainstem, and thalamus) may negatively affect the central mechanisms responsible for the overall system output, which again may influence the perception of fatigue and lead to a disabling feeling of constant exhaustion.[3,5,9]

Cortical Stimulation Studies in Fatigue

Neurophysiologic attempts to identify a CNS source of fatigue, through electrical or magnetic stimulation of the motor cortex and measurement of the resultant muscle force or electrical response in the muscles,[5] have yielded a wealth of information about the role of central processes in the development of this symptom. The current

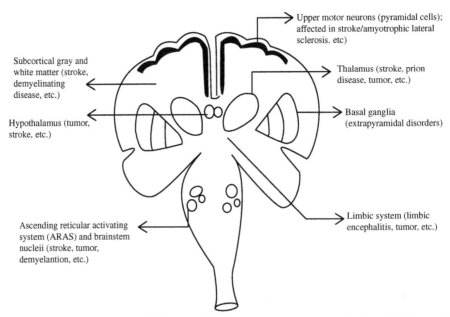

Fig. 3. Various proposed sites of central fatigue, with common causes of central fatigue listed for each site. See text for detailed descriptions. (*Modified from* Chaudhuri A, Behan PO. Fatigue in neurological disorders. Lancet 2004;363(9413):978–88; with permission.)

consensus is that the MVC, recorded in peripheral muscles as described earlier, is submaximal as a result of suboptimal input from supraspinal centers. During the recording of an isometric MVC, twitch amplitudes can be elicited by transcranial magnetic stimulation (TMS) of the motor cortex, suggesting that at least some of the causes of fatigue must lie higher than the motor unit and therefore in the CNS.[10,11] It has also been shown that, after an exhausting task, patients with CNS lesions have a prolonged recovery of TMS-induced motor-evoked potential (MEP) amplitudes, which reflects conduction in the CNS, whereas F-wave latencies and CMAP amplitudes reflecting conduction in the peripheral nervous system were no different from controls. This finding again implicates central conduction pathways in the development of fatigue.[12] In a particularly interesting experiment, Brasil-Neto and colleagues[13] delivered TMS at varying rates after both sustained isometric and isotonic exercise and demonstrated that at 0.3 Hz, a decrement in MEP potential was noted, similar to the phenomenon seen while recording CMAPs with repetitive nerve stimulation (RNS) in postsynaptic neuromuscular junction disorders; this finding has led to the theory that central fatigue might be related at least in part to a reduced safety factor of cortical synaptic transmission in CNS fatigue. Several subsequent experiments have expanded on these findings. Samii and colleagues[14] had 18 normal individuals perform a series of 30-second isometric MVC recordings and consistently showed that after each exercise, TMS-induced MEP amplitudes were, on average, doubled (postexercise facilitation) until fatigue was reached (defined as inability to maintain 50% of MVC), at which point MEP amplitudes produced by TMS were 60% of preexercise baselines (postexercise depression); this recovered over several minutes of rest. These investigators proposed that both postexercise MEP facilitation and MEP depression were caused by intracortical mechanisms. McKay and colleagues[15] showed that the decrease in TMS-induced MEP amplitudes after isometric MVC could not be reproduced after tetanic stimulation of the motor nerve, strongly suggesting that fatigue in this case was caused by failure of the descending motor volley rather than a process at the neuromuscular junction or within the muscle. Other investigators have also determined that the postexercise depression of MEP amplitudes correlates with patients' perception of fatigue, providing evidence of a possible objective measure of a subjective complaint.[16] TMS studies published to date provide evidence of an independent central mechanism for fatigue in patients with CNS disorders, and as the body of literature expands, it is expected that future studies will continue to shed light on the interplay between central and peripheral processes involved in the development of neurologic fatigue.

Common causes of central and peripheral fatigue are listed in **Box 1**.

Physical and Mental Fatigue

Physical fatigue is viewed from a neurologic perspective as the inability to initiate or maintain sustained voluntary activity or force output.[4,9] As previously described, in neurophysiologic terms it is measured as a time-related decline in muscle force generated by MCV[5,17] of muscle force ("SEE SECTION ON PERIPHERAL FATIGUE"). Thus, there is a distinction between physical fatigue and the perception of fatigue; as may be evident from the preceding discussion, one can exist without the other.

A key feature of central fatigue is the presence of both physical and mental fatigue, the latter being defined as a failure to endure sustained mental tasks (eg, mental arithmetic, digit span, remembering a list). In addition, there is a limitation in initiation of action requiring self-motivation, and the overall debilitation is not attributable to abnormal neurologic examination findings (such as motor weakness, coordination difficulty, or sensory loss). This limitation is not a feature of peripheral fatigue, in which there is neurophysiologically demonstrable weakness and a lack of mental fatigue. The term neurasthenia has been used to describe the sum total of the signs and symptoms of central fatigue, especially in CFS, which is the prototype of these disorders.[4] In addition, patients with central fatigue perceive greater expenditure of effort in completing a task, even in the absence of deficits that would limit them from performing the task, and even if the task is completed successfully. Although subjective by its nature, the mental component of central fatigue can be assessed by cognitive and motor-task processing parameters.[9]

MEASURING FATIGUE

Quantification of fatigue between patients, and even in the same patient over time to determine progression and response to therapy, is also challenging, because different patients mean different things when asked to rate their fatigue. Attempts have been made to develop self-reporting fatigue scales for clinical use, and the most widely used include the Checklist Individual Strength[18] and the Abbreviated Fatigue Questionnaire,[19,20] with proven validity and reliability. These questionnaires have been found to be invaluable tools in fatigue-related research. Another commonly used clinical tool is the Fatigue Severity Scale (FSS) (**Box 2**),

Box 1
Major categories of neurologic disorders causing central and peripheral fatigue

Central Fatigue
- Stroke/cerebrovascular disease
- CNS vasculitis
- Granulomatous disease (eg, neurosarcoidosis)
- Demyelinating diseases (eg, MS)
- Extrapyramidal disorders (eg, PD, multiple system atrophy, progressive supranuclear palsy)
- Infectious disease (meningitis/encephalitis)
- Primary sleep disorders (eg, obstructive sleep apnea [OSA], narcolepsy)
- Paraneoplastic diseases (eg, limbic encephalitis, paraneoplastic cerebellitis)
- Idiopathic (CFS)

Peripheral fatigue
- Neuromuscular junction disorders (myasthenia gravis, Lambert-Eaton myasthenic syndrome [LEMS], botulism)
- Channelopathies (eg, periodic paralyses)
- Myopathies, inflammatory (eg, inclusion body myositis, polymyositis/dermatomyositis), drug-induced (statin myopathy, steroid myopathy), metabolic (eg, hypothyroidism, glycogen storage diseases)
- Spinal muscular atrophy
- Charcot-Marie-Tooth disease

Both central and peripheral fatigue
- Infectious disease (eg, neuroborreliosis, neurosyphilis)
- Amyotrophic lateral sclerosis (ALS)
- Post-Guillain Barré syndrome (GBS)/chronic inflammatory demyelinating polyneuropathy
- Mitochondrial diseases
- Myotonic dystrophies
- Postpolio syndrome (PPS)

Box 2
Fatigue Severity Scale (FSS)

Patients choose a number from 1 to 7 that shows their degree of agreement with every statement, where 1 indicates "strongly disagree" and 7 indicates "strongly agree".

- My motivation is lower when I am fatigued
- Exercise brings on my fatigue
- I am easily fatigued
- Fatigue interferes with my physical functioning
- Fatigue causes frequent problems for me
- My fatigue prevents sustained physical functioning
- Fatigue interferes with performing certain duties and responsibilities
- Fatigue is among my 3 most disabling symptoms
- Fatigue interferes with my work, family, or social life

wherein patients choose a rating from 1 to 7 for 9 questions assessing the level of their fatigue. This scale was found to be highly internally consistent and able to distinguish patients with chronic fatigue from controls, as well as to distinguish fatigue in systemic lupus erythematosus (SLE) from those with MS.[21] Part of the problem that researchers of fatigue face is the large number of scales that have been developed; whereas many correlate well, certain others are targeted toward select patient subpopulations, rendering direct comparisons inaccurate. In addition, most fatigue questionnaires are heavily weighted toward eliciting levels of mental fatigue, which may only partly be the source of disability in certain neurologic disorders. These factors need to be taken into account when assessing the efficacy of any treatment modality for fatigue.

CAUSES OF FATIGUE

Chronic fatigue is a known accompaniment of several medical disorders. It is the rule, rather than the exception (and often the presenting complaint), in a wide variety of medical conditions like anemia, autoimmune disorders (eg, SLE, sarcoidosis), chronic infectious diseases such as human immunodeficiency virus and Lyme disease, cardiopulmonary disorders (chronic obstructive pulmonary disease, congestive heart failure), rheumatologic disorders like fibromyalgia, and cancers. In addition, it may be a side effect of a wide variety of medications, most commonly β-blockers, anxiolytics (eg, benzodiazepines, barbiturates), antiepileptics (valproic acid, carbamazepine, levetiracetam), antipsychotics, dopaminergics, proton pump inhibitors, chemotherapeutic agents and β interferons (IFNs), to name the most commonly prescribed classes.[3,9] Fatigue is also a frequent complaint in psychiatric disorders such as major depression, and there has been shown to be a high correlation between complaints of fatigue and psychological morbidity, suggesting a large overlap.[3]

In the neurology clinic, chronic fatigue is frequently seen in a multitude of central (eg, MS, PD, poststroke) and peripheral (neuromuscular junction diseases, GBS, postpolio syndrome, myopathies) causes. Central fatigue is the main problem with the CNS diseases. Although it is logical to expect peripheral fatigue in neuromuscular disorders, central fatigue plays a prominent and independent role in several of them, as discussed in greater detail later.

NEUROIMAGING IN FATIGUE

There has been great recent interest in investigating the usefulness of emerging neuroimaging and neurophysiologic markers of central fatigue, in an attempt both to localize the site of the dysfunction as well as to potentially develop a quantitative measure of a subjective complaint. Although neither structural nor functional neuroimaging studies have identified a single anatomic substrate that is the seat of fatigue, interesting results have been published.[22]

Patients with MS, a central demyelinating disorder, have been evaluated with conventional and functional neuroimaging to attempt to discover the cause of fatigue, a symptom virtually universally present in this population. One recent study found cortical atrophy of the parietal lobe on magnetic resonance imaging (MRI) scans of the brain to have the strongest correlation with fatigue.[23] This finding was confirmed by a contemporaneous report that suggested that the cognitive domain of the Modified Fatigue Impact Scale (MFIS) significantly correlated with atrophy of the striatum and with the cortical thickness of the posterior parietal cortex and middle frontal gyrus, whereas the physical domain of the MFIS significantly correlated with striatum volume and superior frontal gyrus cortical thickness.[24] This is a significant observation, because it suggests that physical and cognitive components of fatigue may arise from different areas of the brain, even within the same disease and the same underlying pathophysiologic mechanism.

Positron emission tomography (PET) scans, which measure cerebral perfusion, have shown widespread cerebral hypometabolism[25] as well as selective hypometabolism in the bifrontal and basal gangliar regions[26] in MS. These findings have led to the postulation that fatigue in this disorder is secondary to disruption of cortical-subcortical pathways secondary to white matter disease. Functional MRI studies have similarly implicated various CNS regions in MS-related fatigue. One study used fMRI to compare patients with MS to controls during a 4-minute finger flexion-extension exercise before and after reaching the point of fatigue. The investigators reported that patients with MS showed greater activation in the contralateral primary motor cortex, insula, and cingulate gyrus than controls before fatigue was reached, but whereas controls showed increased activation of precentral gyrus and insula after fatigue, patients did not show any increases in activation, and showed decreased activity in the insula. This finding suggests that fatigued patients require more effort to complete even simple motor tasks, and are unable to increase central activation once fatigue has occurred, possibly contributing to the development of mental fatigue in addition to physical fatigue.[27]

The absence of specific biomarkers and the subjective nature of criteria required for the diagnosis of

CFS (described in greater detail later), has led to intense interest in the role of neuroimaging in its workup.[28] Early studies suggested that patients with CFS had a greater amount of white matter burden than healthy matched controls.[29,30] Lange and colleagues[31] found a greater number of small, frontal T2 signal punctuate hyperintensities on MRIs of the brain in patients with CFS who did not have a concurrent psychiatric disorder compared with those patients with CFS who did; however, when combined, the CFS group was similar to a healthy control group. Greco and colleagues,[32] studying similar groups of patients, noted a similar trend. Although single-photon emission computed tomography (SPECT) studies have revealed perfusion deficits in the frontal and temporal lobes in patients with CFS compared with healthy controls, they were not found to be different from patients with depression[33] In another study, SPECT scanning showed no differences in cerebral blood flow among patients with CFS compared with healthy controls during a cognitive exercise.[34] However, xenon-computed tomography blood flow studies, which measure absolute blood flow, showed that patients with CFS with no concurrent psychiatric disorders had reduced cortical blood flow in the distribution of both right and left middle cerebral arteries, whereas those with concurrent psychiatric disorders had reduced blood flow only in the left middle cerebral artery territory. Patients with CFS as a group had reduced absolute cortical blood flow in broad areas when compared with data from healthy controls.[35] On PET scans, patients with CFS showed a significant hypometabolism in right mediofrontal cortex and brainstem compared with controls; patients with depression who were concurrently studied showed a severe hypometabolism of the medial and upper frontal regions bilaterally, whereas the metabolism of brain stem was normal.[36] These findings were supported by a subsequent report that confirmed a generalized reduction of brain perfusion, with a particular pattern of hypoperfusion of the brainstem, on the PET scans of patients with CFS.[37]

Given these findings, neuroimaging has not reached a point at which it has everyday clinical usefulness in the diagnosis or prognosis of fatigue. Although the body of literature in this area is expanding rapidly, the modality remains largely in the realm of research.

POSTPOLIO FATIGUE

As many as half of patients with a prior history of poliomyelitis develop post-polio syndrome (PPS), manifested by new onset weakness, pain and fatigue several decades after the acute attack. The cause remains unclear but is believed to be secondary to degeneration of the distal terminal branches of enlarged chronic neurogenic units, perhaps as part of a normal aging process, in patients with already poor neuromuscular reserve.[38] The degree of initial weakness during the acute polio attack (reflecting the number of motor units involved) seems to be the best predictor for the development of PPS.[39] Fatigue is common in these patients, and a recent study showed that younger patients with PPS who had shorter polio duration, more pain, and higher body mass index were more fatigued and had a lower quality of life.[40] Significant fatigue has been reported as high as 77% among patients with PPS; polio survivors without PPS have fatigue rates comparable with healthy controls.[41]

Both central and peripheral causes seem to be at play in PPS-related fatigue. Trojan and colleagues[42] found that patients who showed an improvement in jitter on stimulation single-fiber electromyography (s-sEMG) after administration of intravenous edrophonium also experienced a clinical improvement in fatigue when treated with pyridostigmine, which was not noted in patients who did not have a decrease in jitter with edrophonium administration. This finding suggests that in some patients with PPS, an unstable neuromuscular junction may be the cause of peripheral fatigue. Neuropsychological evaluation of patients with PPS has shown defects of attention and information processing, whereas cognitive abilities and verbal memory were unaffected.[43,44] This finding supports the hypothesis that a polio-related impairment of selective attention underlies polio survivors' subjective experience of fatigue and cognitive problems. In another study, investigators reported word-finding difficulties in 37% of patients with PPS and discovered a negative correlation with plasma prolactin levels and scores on naming tests; the investigators hypothesized that low dopamine levels might be playing a role in this particular symptom.[45] One small study[46] looking at cerebral neuroimaging in PPS found white matter hyperintensities in the reticular formation, putamen, medial leminiscus, and white matter tracts of 55% of patients with PPS with high levels of fatigue, compared with 0% in those with low levels of fatigue. The presence of these lesions correlated with fatigue severity and subjective problems in attention, concentration, and recent memory.

Analysis of sleep dysfunction among patients with PPS has shown a consistent trend of negative impact on sleep continuity. A variety of abnormal movements in sleep, including myoclonus, ballismus, and periodic limb movements of sleep (PLMS) have been reported, possibly affecting sleep quality.[47] PLMS in particular are common in patients with PPS[48] and have a deleterious effect on total sleep time, sleep efficiency, and arousal index. Hypersomnolence caused by sleep-related breathing dysfunction is frequently reported, and these patients have OSA, hypoventilation, or a combination of both.[49]

Patients with PPS experience fatigue daily, and it worsens as the day progresses. Early data seemed to suggest that exercise exacerbated fatigue; in one study, 48% of patients with PPS had worsening of their fatigue with mild exercise, whereas 70% of healthy controls stated that it improved their fatigue.[50] One older study[51] recommended energy conservation and simplification of work skills along with frequent rest periods as a means to combat PPS fatigue. There has been much debate about whether exercise can worsen the rate of motor unit loss, the so-called overuse effect. However, a low-intensity, alternate-day, 12-week quadriceps muscle-strengthening exercise program was evaluated in 12 patients with PPS who showed improvement of physical endurance with no worsening of neurophysiologic parameters or creatine kinase levels.[52] These observations were subsequently confirmed by other investigators.[53] Thus, medically supervised and graded exercise seems to be beneficial in strength preservation in PPS, although the improvement in fatigue scores, if any, remains to be clarified. A study analyzing the relative impact of exercise therapy and cognitive behavioral therapy (CBT) on fatigue in PPS is currently recruiting participants.[54]

With regards to pharmacologic therapy for PPS-related fatigue, multiple agents have been studied. No significant benefit was found with the use of amantadine, an antiviral medication with dopaminergic and activating properties.[55] However, a small trial suggested that bromocriptine, another dopamine agonist used in the treatment of PD, might be efficacious in alleviating all aspects of PPS fatigue, including mental fatigue.[56] Two recent studies have concluded that modafinil, a novel wakefulness-promoting agent with unclear mechanism of action used to treat the excessive daytime sleepiness of narcolepsy, did not show superiority over placebo in alleviating fatigue or improving quality of life.[57,58] Similarly, intravenous immunoglobulin (IVIG), an immunomodulatory agent,[59] has not proved to be of benefit in treating PPS-related fatigue, although it does seem to modestly improve pain. Despite the findings of Trojan and colleagues[60] (see earlier discussion) of improved fatigue with pyridostigmine in patients with PPS who had decreased jitter on s-sEMG with intravenous edrophonium administration, larger studies have not found a benefit.

FATIGUE IN NEUROMUSCULAR JUNCTION DISORDERS

Failure of transmission across the neuromuscular junction is the best-known and most easily studied form of peripheral fatigue. These disorders are routinely evaluated electrophysiologically by RNS studies. CMAPs, obtained by stimulating motor nerves and recording the summated depolarization in supplied muscle fibers, are low at baseline in presynaptic neuromuscular junction diseases such as botulism and Lambert-Eaten myasthenic syndrome. Slow RNS at 3 Hz brings about a decrement (defined as a 10% difference in CMAP amplitude between the highest and the lowest values). Tetanic stimulation (at 50–60 Hz), or sustained voluntary contraction for 10 seconds causes enhanced neuromuscular junction transmission as a result of accumulation of presynaptic intracellular calcium, and at least a 100% increase in CMAP amplitude. In postsynaptic neuromuscular junction disorders like myasthenia gravis, CMAP amplitudes are normal at baseline but slow RNS brings about a U-shaped decrement, which is repaired by tetanic stimulation or 10 seconds of voluntary contraction.[61] Clinically, patients with myasthenia gravis describe a progressive weakness that is partially relieved by rest, although most have bulbar involvement that aids diagnosis. Although the cause and functional limitations of the underlying neuromuscular disease are obvious, fatigue in myasthenia gravis remains a major problem; studies have shown that patients with myasthenia gravis experience significantly more cognitive and physical fatigue than do control individuals, and the patients' perceptions of this fatigue increase significantly after completion of demanding cognitive work.[62]

FATIGUE IN ALS

ALS is characterized by degeneration of upper and lower motor neurons, in the motor cortex and the anterior horn cells of the spinal cord, respectively, leading to a pattern of both upper and lower motor neuron weakness. Patients with ALS commonly complain of fatigue, with the prevalence as high as 83% in some studies, more frequent in younger patients, tending to worsen as the disease progresses,[63] and associated with poorer quality of life.[64] Patients with ALS showed evidence of CAF on MVC studies, as well as less intramuscular phosphocreatine depletion and less fatigue of stimulated tetanic force during exercise compared with controls, suggesting that central fatigue plays a major role in this condition.[65] MVC studies calculating fatigue indices have documented that fatigue is present in muscles not overtly weak, and thus seems to be an independent entity in patients with ALS, distinct from the degree of motor weakness caused by degeneration of upper and lower motor neurons.[66] ALS seems therefore to be an example of a disorder in which both central and peripheral fatigue play significant roles. Probably because of the central component, modafanil has been found to be a promising treatment modality in these patients.[67]

FATIGUE IN NEUROPATHIES AND MYOPATHIES

Many other neuromuscular disorders are associated with fatigue. Fatigue is a common problem in patients with various neuropathies. In a recent study of patients with acquired immune-mediated neuropathies (history of GBS, stable chronic inflammatory demyelinating polyradiculoneuropathy [CIDP] or monoclonal gammopathy-related neuropathy), up to 86% of patients complained of severe fatigue that they found disabling, often persisting years after recovery or stabilization of their symptoms.[68] The mechanism of persistent fatigue in patients who have recovered from GBS may be predominantly central, based on data from analysis of MCV-generated force and CAF.[69] Nerve conduction studies in these patients have failed to show that residual neurophysiologic abnormalities are related to fatigue.[70] Studies in patients with GBS with postrecovery fatigue show no correlation between fatigue severity and the extent of impairment during the acute phase. Similarly, the severity of fatigue does not depend on time between evaluation and recovery from GBS, although fatigue has been shown to be more common in women and patients older than 50 years.[71] A 12-week bicycle exercise training program has resulted in improved fatigue scores in patients with both GBS and CIDP and was well tolerated,[72] suggesting that medically supervised home exercise programs may be beneficial in these patients.[73] Amantadine was found to be of no benefit in post-GBS fatigue,[74] although one case series described modafanil as being useful in alleviating fatigue in patients with hereditary motor and sensory neuropathy type 1 (also known as Charcot-Marie-Tooth 1 disease), the most common inherited neuropathy.[75]

Fatigue is often the presenting symptom in metabolic myopathies, and patients complain of cramping, painful contractions, and myalgias after exercise, while being asymptomatic at rest. This exercise intolerance may occur in the absence of motor weakness or clinical examination abnormalities. Although EMG may be helpful in identifying a myopathic pattern, diagnosis often requires muscle biopsy or genetic testing. Ischemic forearm exercise testing may help distinguish a metabolic block in the glycogenolytic or glycolytic pathway, as seen in McArdle disease, from myoadenylate deficiency; whereas in normal individuals, both ammonia and lactate levels increase in venous blood after exercise, only ammonia increases in the former and only lactate increases in the latter. Extraocular muscle and diaphragmatic involvement, in addition to cerebral white matter changes and varying degrees of encephalopathy, may provide clues to mitochondrial myopathies.[61] Fatigue has also been described in many patients with a variety of inherited myopathies like facioscapulohumeral dystrophy and myotonic dystrophy.[76] Patients with myotonic dystrophy type 1 (DM-1), in particular, have a variety of sleep-related complaints, including sleep-disordered breathing, numerous microarousals, and periodic limb movements. Both fatigue and excessive daytime somnolence are common (76% and 52%, respectively, in one study).[77] Patients with DM-1 with fatigue had more neurologic deficits, longer abnormal triple nucleotide repeats, more psychiatric involvement, and lower quality of life regardless of the presence of excessive daytime sleepiness. However, fatigue and excessive daytime somnolence tended to coexist and it has not yet been possible to separate them out as independent symptoms; this situation argues for aggressive workup and treatment of sleep disorders in this group of patients.

Patients with a group of inherited disorders known as the periodic paralyses, caused by mutations in genes encoding components of membrane ion channels, present with paroxysmal attacks of periodic generalized weakness as well as muscle fatigability brought on by exposure to cold, carbohydrate-rich meals, exercise, or rest, depending on the disorder. Examples for this class of disorder include hypokalemic and hyperkalemic periodic paralysis, myotonia congenita, paramyotonia congenital, and Anderson-Tawil syndrome. Except for the first mentioned, these patients also have myotonia on EMG and can be diagnosed by genetic testing. The duration of muscle weakness is variable in these disorders and may last from a few minutes to a few hours per attack, with a normal neurologic examination, including normal strength testing, in between the attacks. As a class, these disorders tend to be responsive to treatment with acetazolamide, although the mechanism of action of this agent in these conditions is unknown.[61]

A summary of treatment modalities available for peripheral fatigue is provided in **Table 1**.

Table 1
Treatment modalities for common neuromuscular disorders causing peripheral fatigue

Disorder	Treatment
Motor neuron diseases (eg, ALS, spinal muscular atrophy	Supportive care, nocturnal noninvasive positive pressure ventilation in those with nocturnal hypoventilation or evidence of respiratory failure has been proved to prolong life in ALS, riluzole is approved by the US Food and Drug Administration in treatment of ALS
Inflammatory neuropathies (GBS, CIDP)	Immunosuppression (IVIG, plasma exchange; steroids efficacious in treatment of CIDP but not GBS, azathioprine used in CIDP), physical therapy
Inflammatory myopathies (polymyositis/dermatomyositis)	Immunosuppression (steroids therapy), physical therapy
Muscular dystrophies	Supportive care, nocturnal ventilatory support in patients with evidence of respiratory failure
Channelopathies (eg, periodic paralyses)	Acetazolamide therapy, avoid carbohydrate loads and exposure to cold
PPS	Supportive care, exercise therapy
Neuromuscular junction disorders (myasthenia gravis, LEMS)	Symptomatic therapy (acetylcholinesterase inhibitors in myasthenia gravis and LEMS, aminopyridines in LEMS), thymectomy in selected myasthenic patients, immunosuppression (corticosteroids, IVIG, plasma exchange, azathioprine), treatment of underlying malignancy (usually small cell lung cancer) in LEMS

FATIGUE IN MS

Fatigue is a near universal complaint in MS, with prevalence ranging from 46% to up to 85% in various studies. Many patients recall that fatigue often preceded diagnosis or the occurrence of identifiable neurologic lesions by several years. The impact of fatigue on quality of life and daily functioning in this population, as well as fatigue severity scores, are comparable with patients with CFS, although the latter group of patients have significantly higher somatization scores.[78] Fatigue adds significantly to the morbidity of MS, with most patients describing it as the worst or one of the worst symptoms of their disease.[79] Mental fatigue, in particular, closely correlates to cognitive complaints in patients with MS, although neither physical nor mental fatigue has been shown to affect the testing of mental speed, attention, memory, or executive functioning on formal neuropsychiatric evaluation.[80] Many independent studies have proved that fatigue and depression are independently associated with impaired quality of life in MS, after accounting for physical disability.[81,82] Thus, it is clear that physicians cannot draw conclusions about an MS patient's level of fatigue based

on neurologic dysfunction or neuroimaging burden. As with fatigue as a complaint in general, many of these patients may spend several years with their fatigue untreated or undertreated.

The cause of fatigue in MS remains unclear and is likely multifactorial. Neuroimaging research has yet to identify a single brain region that can be blamed for this symptom ("SEE SECTION ON NEUROIMAGING IN FATIGUE"); it is unlikely that such a precise area exists. One group of investigators found that sympathetic dysfunction resembling a hypoadrenergic orthostatic response correlated with fatigue in MS, raising the possibility that sympathomimetics or fluid therapy may have beneficial effects.[83] Unlike CFS, in which a hyporeactivity of the hypothalamopituitary axis (HPA) has been shown, patients with MS with fatigue show a higher activity of the HPA axis than those without fatigue, as shown by significantly increased adrenocorticotropic hormone concentrations.[84] Circulating proinflammatory cytokine levels are also increased in this subgroup of patients, and these two systems seem to act synergistically in producing fatigue, although some groups have suggested that HPA axis dysfunction is more important in producing the cognitive symptoms of MS.[85] Tumor necrosis factor α mRNA expression is higher in patients with MS with fatigue than in those without, whereas no differences are seen for IFN-γ and interleukin 10 mRNA expression. These findings do tend to implicate the proinflammatory state seen in MS with underlying fatigue, but more work needs to be done in this area.

Neurophysiologically, fatigue in MS has been associated with more anteriorly widespread event-related desynchronization during a movement (indicating hyperactivity during movement execution), and lower postmovement contralateral event-related synchronization (indicating failure of the inhibitory mechanisms intervening after movement termination) compared with normal individuals and patients with MS without fatigue. This finding is consistent with central dysfunction and a central origin of fatigue in MS.[86]

IFN therapy is generally acknowledged as a major contributor to MS-related fatigue, often leading to discontinuation of treatment,[87] although some studies have suggested that it may not play as big a role as previously believed.[88] Glatiramer acetate is effective in treating MS-related fatigue[89] and was found in 1 study to be more beneficial than IFN-β in this outcome measure.[90] Oral levocarnitine administration decreased fatigue intensity, especially in patients treated with cyclophosphamide and IFN-β, in 63% of patients treated with immunomodulatory therapy.[91]

The relationship between MS-related fatigue and sleep disorders has been evaluated as well. It has been shown that although sleep dysfunction, depression, and disease severity were all independent contributors to fatigue in MS, sleep dysfunction was the strongest predictor.[92] Excessive limb movements, nocturia, and pain are the main symptoms resulting in fragmented sleep and poor sleep efficiency in MS. Insomnia is a common complaint, with pain and discomfort being linked to sleep initiation insomnia, and nocturia being linked to sleep maintenance insomnia; the latter had a stronger association with fatigue.[93] One study found that 80% to 96% of patients with MS with fatigue had a sleep disorder, compared with only 20% of nonfatigued patients with MS and 0% of healthy matched controls. The sleep disturbances included delayed sleep phase and sleep disruption, and 60% of the fatigued MS group had Epworth Sleepiness Scale (ESS) scores greater than 10, suggesting significant daytime somnolence. This finding was associated with increased fatigue.[94] In another study, 25% of patients with MS with fatigue had sleep-disordered breathing, compared with 2.5% in the nonfatigued MS group.[95] However, sleep-disordered breathing per se is not believed

to be an explanation for the fatigue in these patients.[96] This early investigative work makes it clear that treating physicians should keep the possibility of a sleep disorder in mind while treating patients with MS complaining of fatigue and consider referral to a sleep center if the history or physical examination suggests that a treatable sleep disorder may be present.

Treatment of fatigue in MS has proved to be challenging. Modafanil has performed unevenly in studies; one study suggested that 200 mg/d was well tolerated and effective in reducing MS-related fatigue,[97,98] but it was found to be no better than placebo in a more recent randomized double-blind study, even at doses twice as large.[99] Nevertheless, it remains a popular and relatively safe drug, with the most common side effect being headache, and is considered first line for MS-related fatigue. Amantadine produced small but statistically significant improvements in fatigue across 4 of 7 dimensions (overall energy level, concentration, problem solving, and sense of well-being) in a double-blind control study. Its long-term efficacy remains unclear.[100] Older studies suggested that the CNS stimulant pemoline may potentially be an effective short-term treatment of fatigue associated with MS, but its adverse effects, including anorexia, irritability, and insomnia, are not well tolerated by many patients. Doses lower than 75 mg/d were less effective, and reports of liver failure have led to a US Food and Drug Administration black box warning.[101] With more recent data suggesting that pemoline is no better than placebo in MS-related fatigue, the medication has more or less fallen out of favor,[102] although individual patients may still benefit from it. Neither amantadine nor pemoline was found to be effective in treating cognitive complaints in MS.[103] Certainly, given the strong coexistence of depression and fatigue in MS, treatment with antidepressants such as selective serotonin reuptake inhibitors (SSRIs), monoamine oxidase inhibitors (MAOIs), tricyclic antidepressants, selective serotonin-norepinephrine reuptake inhibitors, and dopamine-norepinephine reuptake inhibitors should be considered, although there are few systematic studies assessing their efficacy in MS-related fatigue as a separate symptom.

Nonpharmacologic measures for managing fatigue are more consistently beneficial in patients with MS-related fatigue. However, unlike in CFS, treating physicians and physical therapists need to be aware of the patient's neurologic disabilities and the worsening of symptoms with heat exposure. There is a tendency among patients and the medical community to discourage physical activity and exertion in MS, but the literature does not support this recommendation. A progressive

6-month exercise program was found to improve speed of walking in patients with MS, with a program completion rate of 96%.[104] Brief, moderate, aerobic exercise has been repeatedly shown to improve physical fitness in individuals with mild MS, with no evidence of worsening of symptoms in association with exercises.[105] The cumulative evidence supports the theory that exercise training is associated with a small improvement in quality of life among individuals with MS.[106] Similarly, studies comparing CBT and relaxation therapy have found both to be clinically effective treatments for fatigue in patients with MS, although the effects for CBT are greater than those for relaxation therapy. Even 6 months after treatment, both treatment groups reported levels of fatigue equivalent to those of a healthy comparison group.[107] Success rates for CBT seem to be better in MS-related fatigue than in CFS. With Internet usage rapidly expanding worldwide, there has been interest in developing online fatigue self-management Web sites. However, a recent study evaluating the effectiveness of such an online program among patients with MS-related fatigue, PD-related fatigue, and PPS-related fatigue did not show benefit over a control group.[108] Nevertheless, this remains a fertile field for future research. An interesting recent crossover study evaluated exposure to a low-frequency magnetic field, but found no advantage over sham exposure in reducing the impact of fatigue in patients with MS.[109]

POSTSTROKE FATIGUE

Often neglected or overshadowed by the patient's more obvious neurologic deficits, fatigue is nevertheless a common and debilitating feature in poststroke patients. The incidence has been found to be as high as 45%.[110] In a recent 2-year follow-up study,[111] poststroke fatigue levels decreased after 3 months and remained stable throughout the remainder of follow-up. Increased levels of fatigue were consistently associated with poor functional outcome. The same study found that the fatigue was mainly physical; this confirms the observation in other studies that the presence of fatigue was independent of depression. However, the impact of fatigue on functional abilities was strongly influenced by depression.[112] Risk factors for the development of poststroke fatigue seem to be younger age, poststroke depressive symptoms, and infratentorial infarctions.[113] Poststroke fatigue seems to be an independent determinant of not being able to resume paid work after stroke.[114]

Attempts have been made to formulate scales to quantify poststroke fatigue, similar to ones developed for CFS and MS. Lynch and colleagues[115] developed a new case definition for this entity and are awaiting its further evaluation in different clinical settings.

Treatment options for patients with poststroke fatigue remain limited. In a recent double-blind, placebo-controlled trial,[116] fluoxetine was not shown to improve poststroke fatigue, although it was helpful in poststroke emotional incontinence and poststroke depression. Chronic disease self-management programs have also not been found to be helpful. There are no clear guidelines or recommendations for treating poststroke fatigue. The role of CBT and medications like modafinil or amantadine remain uncertain in this setting.[117]

FATIGUE IN PD

Fatigue is a common nonmotor complaint among patients with PD, being a disabling symptom in up to two-thirds of this population.[118] As with MS, fatigue in PD overlaps with depression, but they do not seem to be causally related.[119] Fatigue was highly correlated with poor scores on quality of life indicators, independent of depression and dementia.[120] Patients with PD with more severe fatigue are more sedentary and have poorer functional capacity and physical function compared with patients with less fatigue.[121] As with other causes of central fatigue, the underlying mechanisms for the symptom in PD remain unknown, but functional neuroimaging has suggested that reduced serotonergic function in the basal ganglia and limbic structures may be important. Insular dopaminergic dysfunction could also play a role.[122] Other studies have used SPECT scans to identify frontal lobe dysfunction in fatigued patients with PD.[123] There is also evidence of a peripheral manifestation of PD-related fatigue in the form of muscle fatigability,[124] although this is responsive to dopaminergic therapy and therefore believed to be still central in cause.

Sleep problems play a major role in PD, including insomnia, circadian rhythm abnormalities, restless legs syndrome (RLS)/PLMS, nocturnal bradykinesia and discomfort, complicated sleep apnea, and rapid eye movement (REM) behavior disorder,[125] leading to excessive daytime sleepiness and a narcoleptic phenotype. However, fatigue in PD was found to be independent of excessive daytime sleepiness.[126]

Optimal treatment of fatigue in PD is still unclear, although there is evidence of at least a partial response to levodopa therapy on physical fatigue.[127] Although CBT has been proved to be useful in managing depression in PD, its effects on fatigue have not been systematically analyzed, nor has a graded exercise program.[128]

CFS

CFS (also known as myalgic encephalitis) remains a poorly understood and still controversial diagnosis. Estimates of its prevalence among primary care practices vary widely, ranging from 0.002% to 11.3%.[129,130] Some studies have indicated increased prevalence among women, minority groups, and persons with lower levels of education and occupational status.[131] Significant comorbidity with psychiatric disorders has also been noted.[132,133] However, it has been postulated that the psychological disturbances in these patients are more a consequence of the illness rather than a predisposing factor to it.[134]

Multiple attempts have been made to develop criteria for the diagnosis of this disorder. Although complaints of chronic physical and mental fatigue lasting greater than 6 months without another medical condition to which such symptoms could be attributed is the essential symptom, investigators have struggled to reach a consensus on other required features. In 1994, Fukuda and colleagues[135] proposed a set of guidelines for diagnosing CFS. These guidelines were followed by Centers for Disease Control (CDC) diagnostic criteria published the same year (**Box 3**). Many symptoms included in the criteria remain nebulous and subjective; although the development of these criteria has helped in standardizing the diagnosis of CFS, we remain a long way off from identifying convincing tests or elucidating underlying pathophysiology.

The cause of CFS remains elusive. The concept of a postviral cause remains popular, although no particular organism has been consistently identified.

Many patients complain of relatively acute onset of fatiguing signs and symptoms after a flulike illness. However, seroprevalence of antibodies to herpes simplex virus 1 and 2, rubella, adenovirus, human herpesvirus 6, Epstein-Barr virus, cytomegalovirus, and Coxsackie B virus types 1–6 in patients with CFS was compared with healthy control individuals and no significant differences were found. Assaying these antibodies was not considered fruitful in making a diagnosis of CFS, and no conclusion as to the cause of CFS could be drawn.[136] Enteroviral titers similarly showed no association.[137] There was initial interest in a newly discovered human retrovirus, xenotropic murine leukemia virus-related virus, found to be present in 67% of persons from the United States with CFS by polymerase chain reaction detection.[138] However, subsequent studies have not been able to confirm such an association.[139]

Immune dysfunction is well known in CFS; compared with healthy controls, a reduced CD8 suppressor cell population and increased activation markers (CD38, HLA-DR) on CD8 cells were found, with the differences being significant in patients with more severe disease. No correlation of these findings in patients with CFS with any known human viruses could be detected by serology.[140] Other immunologic changes reported in CFS include cytokine abnormalities and natural killer cell dysfunction. Proinflammatory cytokines were believed to be the cause of the fatigue and flulike symptoms. Abnormal activation of the T-lymphocyte subsets and a decrease in antibody-dependent cell-mediated cytotoxicity have been described. An

---

Box 3
CDC criteria for the diagnosis of CFS

In order to be diagnosed with CFS, a patient must satisfy 2 criteria:

1. Have severe chronic fatigue for at least 6 months or longer with other known medical conditions (whose manifestation includes fatigue) excluded by clinical diagnosis; and

2. Concurrently have 4 or more of the following symptoms:

   a. Postexertional malaise

   b. Impaired memory or concentration

   c. Unrefreshing sleep

   d. Muscle pain

   e. Multijoint pain without redness or swelling

   f. Tender cervical or axillary lymph nodes

   g. Sore throat

   h. Headache

The symptoms must have persisted or recurred during 6 or more consecutive months of illness and must not have predated the fatigue.

increased number of CD8+ cytotoxic T lymphocytes and CD38 and HLA-DR activation markers have been reported, and a decrease in CD11b expression associated with an increased expression of CD28+ T subsets has been observed.[141] These findings suggest that immune activation is associated with many cases of CFS.

It has been clearly shown that the site of dysfunction in CFS is central and not peripheral. Compared with healthy controls, a group of 14 women with CFS were shown to have greater CAF in the first 45 seconds of a 2-minute-long MVC of the biceps brachii muscle, and had less peripheral fatigue as measured by comparisons of stimulation-induced force responses before and after MCV.[142]

In a study comparing neurology clinic patients with a diagnosis of CFS to patients with established peripheral causes (neuromuscular diseases such as ALS, GBS, and genetic or metabolic myopathies) and inpatients with psychiatric diagnoses (major depression, the affective group), mental fatigue was comparable in the CFS and affective group and more significantly prevalent than in the neuromuscular group, whereas there was no significant difference between the groups with respect to physical fatigue as measured by questionnaires. The investigators inferred the central origin of fatigue in CFS from this finding, and also discovered that twice as many patients with CFS met criteria for a psychiatric illness as did patients with neuromuscular disease.[133]

There have been few studies looking at sleep complaints in patients with CFS.[143] One study found a variety of sleep disorders (sleep initiation and maintenance insomnia, excessive time in bed with poor sleep efficiency and hypersomnolence) in patients who met criteria for CFS but not major depressive syndrome, but a cause-and-effect relationship could not be established.[144] When a subset of patients meeting criteria for CFS who self-reported sleep disturbances were studied with polysomnography (PSG), disorders found included OSA, periodic limb movement disorders, and narcolepsy.[145,146] However, it was believed that most patients with CFS had normal PSGs or only had nonspecific abnormalities.[147] When compared with controls, sleep onset latency and slow wave sleep abnormalities were noted, but mean REM onset latency was not significantly different.[148] Alpha-delta sleep was not found to be a marker of CFS.[149] Although comorbid sleep disturbances seem likely in patients with CFS, the paucity of literature in this regard makes this an area ripe for research.

Pharmacologic treatment options for CFS remain particularly unsatisfactory. HPA hypofunction has been implicated in the disease, and low-dose oral hydrocortisone therapy was found to improve Global Wellness Scale scores in patients with CFS compared with controls, but the degree of adrenal suppression was considered unacceptably high.[150] Similarly, although growth hormone therapy was found not to improve quality of life indices, 23% of patients so treated returned to work after long absences.[151] There have been contradictory results with trials of IVIG in the treatment of CFS, although most studies indicate no benefit.[152–154]

CBT has consistently been found effective in CFS.[155,156] In one study,[157] the investigators noted that patient outcome depended more on the strength of the initial attribution of symptoms by the patient to exclusively physical causes, and was not influenced by length of illness. However, a more recent study[158] suggested that beliefs about the physical nature of the illness did not affect effectiveness of CBT as much as was previously believed. CBT was found to be more effective than guided control groups[159] and was determined to be superior to relaxation therapy in a 5-year follow-up study, with more than 80% of patients still using it at the end of the study.[160] It was also proven to be particularly effective in a subset of patients who had CFS with cognition-related depressive signs and symptoms.[161] A recent study also suggested that CBT may increase prefrontal cortical volume in patients with CFS.[162] Low-impact, graded aerobic exercise therapy was also found to be a beneficial strategy,[163] especially when combined with patient education about the underlying physiologic mechanisms for fatigue.[164] Physicians and physical therapists have been advised to counsel patients with chronic fatigue to concentrate on regularity of exercise, rather than the result of such activity. Although there is clearly a need for more long-term studies, these nonpharmacologic techniques of combating fatigue seem more promising in improving quality of life in patients with CFS and chronic fatigue from any cause.[165] It has been recommended that medical retirement should be postponed until a trial of such treatment has been given.[166] Fluoxetine, an SSRI, was found to be ineffective in treating the nondepressive features of CFS, and inferior to graded exercise therapy in this regard.[167,168]

The natural history of CFS remains to be elucidated. Medium-term studies have been equivocal. One study[169] found poor recovery, with illness duration, mode of onset, psychiatric status, and chemical sensitivity not predicting outcome. However, other studies have suggested that older patients, those with psychiatric comorbidities, longer illness duration, and a belief that their symptoms are physical rather than psychological do worse in terms of recovery. Return to premorbid level of functioning was better in children and those with fatigue of less than 6 months' duration (although the latter group would not meet criteria for CFS).[170] While the incidence of chronic fatigue and CFS in adolescents aged 11 to 15 years was comparable with the adult population, the prognosis was considered good, in contrast to the dismal outcome in adults.[171,172]

FATIGUE IN PRIMARY SLEEP DISORDERS

OSA, a disorder of repetitive breathing disturbances in sleep caused by partial reversible airway obstruction leading to fragmented sleep, is commonly associated with fatigue, and, as with MS, is strongly correlated with but independent of depression. Up to 42% of patients with OSA complain of fatigue, and research has suggested that increased body weight and higher levels of proinflammatory cytokines may play a role.[173] However, the level of fatigue does not seem to be related to the severity of OSA as measured by the degree of event-related hypoxemia,[174] and fatigue scores do not correlate with objective measures of daytime sleepiness such as the mean sleep latency on the multiple sleep latency test, suggesting that excessive daytime somnolence and fatigue in OSA are separate symptoms with different causes.[175] Nevertheless, increasing sleep fragmentation, as measured by the arousal index on the PSG, did worsen self-reported fatigue.[176] Treatment of OSA with continuous positive airway pressure (CPAP) has been proved to improve fatigue; in 1 study, 3 weeks of CPAP therapy significantly improved both excessive daytime sleepiness and fatigue scores.[177] Although the exact prevalence is unclear, fatigue is also commonly seen in narcolepsy, a primary sleep disorder characterized by poor nocturnal sleep quality, excessive daytime somnolence and intrusion of rapid eye movement (REM) phenomena into wakefulness. One study found severe fatigue in 63% of narcoleptics with cataplexy, whereas ESS scores were comparable among participants who complained of fatigue and those who did not, again suggesting that fatigue and excessive daytime sleepiness are separate symptoms[178] Modafinil, which is commonly used to treat the excessive daytime somnolence seen with this disorder, has also been shown to improve fatigue and quality of life indicators in a group of patients switched from psychostimulants.[179] Patients with RLS and PLMS, motor disorders that may cause insomnia and disrupt sleep, often complain of fatigue as well, although systematic study of this complaint in these patients is sparse. However, in one study,[180] patients with type 2 diabetes and RLS had significantly higher FSS scores than patients without RLS. A recent report suggests that PLMS may contribute to daytime fatigue in patients with motor sequelae of polio.[181]

SUMMARY

Fatigue is a common complaint and a major source of disability for patients with neurologic diseases. Fatigue must be distinguished as a separate symptom from weakness, muscle fatigability, depression, and excessive daytime sleepiness, because it often requires a different management strategy. In most neurologic disorders, both central and peripheral fatigue play a role in the patient's disability. Fatigue is independent of neurologic disability and depression and is often limiting, with a significant impact on quality of life. Research into neuroimaging findings in fatigue remains in its infancy. Although various pharmacologic agents have been tried to treat fatigue in a variety of disorders, for most patients with central fatigue, a combination of CBT and a graded exercise program seems to be most efficacious. It is crucial that health care providers regularly enquire into the presence and adequate treatment of fatigue in their patients.

REFERENCES

1. Victor M, Ropper AH, editors. Adams and Victor's principles of neurology. 7th edition. New York: McGraw-Hill; 2001.
2. Pawlikowska T, Chalder T, Hirsch SR, et al. Population based study of fatigue and psychological distress. BMJ 1994;308:763–6.
3. Krupp LB. Fatigue. Philadelphia: Butterworth-Heinemann; 2003.
4. Chaudhuri A, Behan PO. Fatigue and basal ganglia. J Neurol Sci 2000;179(1–2):34–42.
5. Zwarts MJ, Bleijenberg G, van Engelen BG. Clinical neurophysiology of fatigue. Clin Neurophysiol 2008;119:2–10.
6. Kent-Braun J. Central and peripheral contributions to muscle fatigue in humans during sustained maximal effort. Eur J Appl Physiol 1999;80:57–63.
7. Holmes G, Kaplan J, Gantz N, et al. Chronic fatigue syndrome: a working case definition. Ann Intern Med 1988;108:387–9.
8. Grandjean E. Fatigue in industry. Br J Ind Med 1979;36:175–86.
9. Chaudhuri A, Behan PO. Fatigue in neurological disorders. Lancet 2004;363(9413):978–88.
10. Gandevia SC, Allen GM, Butler JE, et al. Supraspinal factors in human muscle fatigue: evidence for suboptimal output from the motor cortex. J Physiol 1996;490:529–36.

11. Taylor JL, Gandevia SC. Transcranial magnetic stimulation and human muscle fatigue. Muscle Nerve 2001;24:18–29.

12. Liepert J, Kotterba S, Tegenthoff M, et al. Central fatigue assessed by transcranial magnetic stimulation. Muscle Nerve 1996;19:1429–34.

13. Brasil-Neto JP, Cohen LG, Hallett M. Central fatigue as revealed by postexercise decrement of motor evoked potentials. Muscle Nerve 1994;17:713–9.

14. Samii A, Wassermann EM, Ikoma K, et al. Characterization of postexercise facilitation and depression of motor evoked potentials to transcranial magnetic stimulation. Neurology 1996;46(5):1376–82.

15. McKay WB, Tuel SM, Sherwood AM, et al. Focal depression of cortical excitability induced by fatiguing muscle contraction: a transcranial magnetic stimulation study. Exp Brain Res 1995;105(2):276–82.

16. Brasil-Neto JP, Pascual-Leone A, Valls-Sole J, et al. Postexercise depression of motor evoked potentials: a measure of central nervous system fatigue. Exp Brain Res 1993;93(1):181–4.

17. Bigland-Ritchie B, Jones DA, Hosking GP. Central and peripheral fatigue in sustained maximum voluntary contractions of human quadriceps muscle. Clin Sci Mol Med 1978;54:609–14.

18. Beurskens AJ, Bultmann U, Kant I, et al. Fatigue among working people: validity of a questionnaire measure. Occup Environ Med 2000;57:353–7.

19. Albers M, Smets EM, Vercoulen JH, et al. Abbreviated fatigue questionnaire; a practical tool in the classification of fatigue. Ned Tijdschr Geneeskd 1997;141:1526–30 [in Dutch].

20. Albers M, Vercoulen JH, Bleijenberg G. Assessment of fatigue. The practical utility of the subjective feeling of fatigue in research and clinical practice. In: Vingerhoets A, editor. Assessment in behavioral medicine. Brunner (New Zealand): Routledge; 2001. p. 301–27.

21. Krupp L, LaRocca N, Muir-Nash J, et al. The fatigue severity scale: application to patients with multiple sclerosis and systemic lupus erythematosus. Arch Neurol 1989;46(10):1121–3.

22. DeLuca J, Genova H, Capili E, et al. Functional neuroimaging of fatigue. Phys Med Rehabil Clin N Am 2009;20(2):325–37.

23. Pellicano C, Gallo A, Li X. Relationship of cortical atrophy to fatigue in patients with multiple sclerosis. Arch Neurol 2010;67(4).447–53.

24. Calabrese M, Rinaldi F, Grossi P, et al. Basal ganglia and frontal/parietal cortical atrophy is associated with fatigue in relapsing-remitting multiple sclerosis. Mult Scler 2010;16(10):1220–8.

25. Bakshi R, Miletich RS, Kinkel PR, et al. High-resolution fluorodeoxyglucose positron emission tomography shows both global and regional cerebral hypometabolism in multiple sclerosis. J Neuroimaging 1998;8: 228–34.

26. Roelcke U, Kappos L, Lechner-Scott J, et al. Reduced glucose metabolism in the frontal cortex and basal ganglia of multiple sclerosis patients with fatigue: a 18F-fluorodeoxyglucose positron emission tomography study. Neurology 1997;48: 1566–71.

27. White AT, Lee JN, Light AR, et al. Brain activation in multiple sclerosis: a BOLD fMRI study of the effects of fatiguing hand exercise. Mult Scler 2009;15(5): 580–6.

28. Lange G, Wang S, DeLuca J, et al. Neuroimaging in chronic fatigue syndrome. Am J Med 1998; 105(3A):50S–3S.

29. Natelson BH, Cohen JM, Brassloff I, et al. A controlled study of brain magnetic resonance imaging in patients with the chronic fatigue syndrome. J Neurol Sci 1993;120:213–7.

30. Cope H, Pernet A, Kendall B, et al. Cognitive functioning and magnetic resonance imaging in chronic fatigue syndrome. Br J Psychiatry 1995;167:86–94.

31. Lange G, DeLuca J, Maldjian J, et al. Brain MRI abnormalities exist in a subset of patients with chronic fatigue syndrome. J Neurol Sci 1999;17(1):3–7.

32. Greco A, Tannock C, Brostoff J, et al. Brain MR in chronic fatigue syndrome. AJNR Am J Neuroradiol 1997;18(7):1265–9.

33. Schwartz RB, Komaroff AL, Garada BM, et al. SPECT imaging of the brain: comparison of findings in patients with chronic fatigue syndrome, AIDS dementia complex, and major unipolar depression. AJR Am J Roentgenol 1994;162(4):943–51.

34. Schmaling K, Lewis D, Fiedelak J, et al. Single-photon emission computerized tomography and neurocognitive function in patients with chronic fatigue syndrome. Psychosom Med 2003;65:129–36.

35. Yoshiuchi K, Farkas J, Natelson BH. Patients with chronic fatigue syndrome have reduced absolute cortical blood flow. Clin Physiol Funct Imaging 2006;26:83–6.

36. Tirelli U, Chierichetti F, Tavio M, et al. Brain positron emission tomography (PET) in chronic fatigue syndrome: preliminary data. Am J Med 1998; 105(3 Suppl 1):54S–8S.

37. Costa DC, Tannocki C, Brostoff J. Brainstem perfusion is impaired in chronic fatigue syndrome. QJM 1995;88(11):767–73.

38. Trojan DA, Cashman NR. Post-poliomyelitis syndrome. Muscle Nerve 2005;31:6–19.

39. Trojan DA, Cashman NR, Shapiro S, et al. Predictive factors for post-poliomyelitis syndrome. Arch Phys Med Rehabil 1994;75(7):770–7.

40. Östlund G, Wahlin Å, Sunnerhagen KS, et al. Post polio syndrome: fatigued patients a specific subgroup? J Rehabil Med 2011;43(1):39–45.

41. On AY, Oncu J, Atamaz F, et al. Impact of post-polio fatigue on quality of life. J Rehabil Med 2006;38:329–32.

42. Trojan DA, Genrdon D, Cashman NR. Anticholines-terase-responsive neuromuscular junction transmission defects in post-poliomyelitis fatigue. J Neurol Sci 1993;114(2):170–7.

43. Bruno RL, Galski T, DeLuca J. The neuropsychology of post-polio fatigue. Arch Phys Med Rehabil 1993; 74(10):1061–5.

44. Ostlund G, Borg K, Wahlin A. Cognitive functioning in post-polio patients with and without general fatigue. J Rehabil Med 2005;37(3):147–51.

45. Bruno RL, Zimmerman JR. Word finding difficulty as a post-polio sequelae. Am J Phys Med Rehabil 2000;79(4):343–8.

46. Bruno RL, Cohen JM, Frick NM. The neuroanatomy of post-polio fatigue. Arch Phys Med Rehabil 1994; 75:498–504.

47. Bruno R. Abnormal movements in sleep as a post-polio sequelae. Am J Phys Med Rehabil 1998; 77(4):339–43.

48. Araujo MA, de Silva TM, Moreira GA, et al. Sleep disorders frequency in post-polio syndrome patients caused by periodic limb movements. Arq Neuropsiquiatr 2010;68(1):35–8.

49. Hsu AA, Staats BA. "Postpolio" sequelae and sleep-related disordered breathing. Mayo Clin Proc 1998;73(3):216–24.

50. Berlly MH, Strauser WW, Hall KM. Fatigue in post-polio syndrome. Arch Phys Med Rehabil 1991; 72(2):115–8.

51. Packer TL, Martins I, Krefting L. Activity and post-polio fatigue. Orthopedics 1991;14(11):1223–6.

52. Agre J, Rodriguez A, Franke T, et al. Low-intensity, alternate-day exercise improves muscle performance without apparent adverse affect in postpolio patients. Am J Phys Med Rehabil 1996;75(1):50–8.

53. Chan KM, Amirjani N, Sumrain M, et al. Randomized controlled trial of strength training in post-polio patients. Muscle Nerve 2003;27:332–8.

54. Koopman FS, Beelen A, Gerrits KH, et al. Exercise therapy and cognitive behavioural therapy to improve fatigue, daily activity performance and quality of life in postpoliomyelitis syndrome: the protocol of the FACTS-2-PPS trial. BMC Neurol 2010;18(10):8.

55. Stein DP, Dambrosia JM, Dalakas MC. A double-blind, placebo-controlled, trial of amantadine for the treatment, of fatigue in patients with the post-polio syndrome. Ann N Y Acad Sci 1998;753:296–302.

56. Bruno R, Zimmerman J, Creange S, et al. Bromocriptine in the treatment of post-polio fatigue: a pilot study with implications for the pathophysiology of fatigue. Am J Phys Med Rehabil 1996;75(5):340–7.

57. Chan KM, Strohschein FJ, Rydz D, et al. Randomized controlled trial of modafinil for the treatment of fatigue in postpolio patients. Muscle Nerve 2006; 33:138–41.

58. Vasconcelos OM, Prokhorenko OA, Salajegheh MK, et al. Modafinil for treatment of fatigue in post-polio syndrome: a randomized controlled trial. Neurology 2007;68(20):1680–6.

59. Farbu E, Rekand T, Vik-Mo E, et al. Post-polio syndrome patients treated with intravenous immunoglobulin: a double-blinded randomized controlled pilot study. Eur J Neurol 2007;14:60–5.

60. Trojan DA, Collet JP, Shapiro S, et al. A multicenter, randomized, double-blinded trial of pyridostigmine in postpolio syndrome. Neurology 1999;53(6): 1225–33.

61. Preston DC, Shapiro BE, editors. Electromyography and neuromuscular disorders: clinical-electrophysiological correlates. 2nd edition. Philadelphia: Elsevier Butterworth-Heinemann; 2005.

62. Paul RH, Cohen RA, Goldstein JM, et al. Fatigue and its impact on patients with myasthenia gravis. Muscle Nerve 2000;23:1402–6.

63. Ramirez C, Piemonte ME, Callegaro D, et al. Fatigue in amyotrophic lateral sclerosis: frequency and associated factors. Amyotroph Lateral Scler 2008;9(2):75–80.

64. Lou JS, Reeves A, Benice T, et al. Fatigue and depression are associated with poor quality of life in ALS. Neurology 2003;60(1):122–3.

65. Kent-Braun JA, Miller RG. Central fatigue during isometric exercise in amyotrophic lateral sclerosis. Muscle Nerve 2000;23:909–14.

66. Sanjak M, Brinkmann J, Beldon DS, et al. Quantitative assessment of motor fatigue in amyotrophic lateral sclerosis. J Neurol Sci 2001;191(1):55–9.

67. Rabkin JG, Gordon PH, McElhiney M, et al. Modafinil treatment of fatigue in patients with ALS: a placebo-controlled study. Muscle Nerve 2009;39: 297–303.

68. Merkies IS, Schmitz PI, Samijn JP, et al. Fatigue in immune-mediated polyneuropathies. Neurology 1999;53(8):1648–54.

69. Garssen MP, Schillings ML, Van Doorn PA, et al. Contribution of central and peripheral factors to residual fatigue in Guillain-Barré syndrome. Muscle Nerve 2007;36:93–9.

70. Garssen MP, van Doorn PA, Visser GH. Nerve conduction studies in relation to residual fatigue in Guillain-Barré syndrome. J Neurol 2006;253(7): 851–6.

71. Garssen MP, van Koningsveld R, Van Doorn PA. Residual fatigue is independent of antecedent events and disease severity in Guillain-Barré syndrome. J Neurol 2006;253(9):1143–6.

72. Garssen MP, Busmann JB, Scmitz PI, et al. Physical training and fatigue, fitness, and quality of life in Guillain-Barré syndrome and CIDP. Neurology 2004;63(12):2393–5.

73. Ruhland JL, Shields RK. The effects of a home exercise program on impairment and health-related quality of life in persons with chronic peripheral neuropathies. Phys Ther 1997;77(10):1026–39.

74. Garssen MP, Schmitz PI, Merlies IS, et al. Amantadine for treatment of fatigue in Guillain-Barré syndrome: a randomised, double blind, placebo controlled, crossover trial. J Neurol Neurosurg Psychiatry 2006;77:61–5.

75. Carter G, Han J, Mayadev A. Modafinil reduces fatigue in Charcot-Marie-Tooth disease type 1a: a case series. Am J Hosp Palliat Care 2006;23(5):412–6.

76. Kalkman JS, Schillings ML, van der Werf SP, et al. Experienced fatigue in facioscapulohumeral dystrophy, myotonic dystrophy, and HMSN-1. J Neurol Neurosurg Psychiatry 2005;76(10):1406–9.

77. Salva MQ, Blumen M, Jacquette A, et al. Sleep disorders in childhood-onset myotonic dystrophy type 1. Neuromuscul Disord 2006;16(9–10):564–70.

78. Vercoulen JH, Hommes OR, Swanink C, et al. The measurement of fatigue in patients with multiple sclerosis: a multidimensional comparison with patients with chronic fatigue syndrome and healthy subjects. Arch Neurol 1996;53(7):642–9.

79. Fisk JD, Pontefract A, Ritvo PG, et al. The impact of fatigue on patients with multiple sclerosis. Can J Neurol Sci 1994;21(1):9–14.

80. Bol Y, Duits AA, Hupperts RM, et al. The impact of fatigue on cognitive functioning in patients with multiple sclerosis. Clin Rehabil 2010;24(9):854–62.

81. Janardhana V, Bakshi R. Quality of life in patients with multiple sclerosis: the impact of fatigue and depression. J Neurol Sci 2002;205(1):51–8.

82. Amato MP, Ponziani G, Rossi F, et al. Quality of life in multiple sclerosis: the impact of depression, fatigue and disability. Mult Scler 2001;7(5):340–4.

83. Flachenecker P, Rufer A, Bihler I, et al. Fatigue in MS is related to sympathetic vasomotor dysfunction. Neurology 2003;61(6):851–3.

84. Gottschalk M, Kümpfel T, Flachenecker P, et al. Fatigue and regulation of the hypothalamo-pituitary-adrenal axis in multiple sclerosis. Arch Neurol 2005;62:277–80.

85. Heesen C, Nawrath L, Reich C, et al. Fatigue in multiple sclerosis: an example of cytokine mediated sickness behaviour? J Neurol Neurosurg Psychiatry 2006;77:34–9.

86. Leocani L, Colombo B, Magnani G, et al. Fatigue in multiple sclerosis is associated with abnormal cortical activation to voluntary movement–EEG evidence. Neuroimage 2001;13(6 Pt 1):1186–92.

87. Nielly L, Goodin D, Goodkin D, et al. Side effect profile of interferon beta-1b in MS: results of an open label trial. Neurology 1996;46:552–3.

88. Putzki N, Katsarava Z, Vago S, et al. Prevalence and severity of multiple-sclerosis-associated fatigue in treated and untreated patients. Eur Neurol 2008;59:136–42.

89. Ziemssen T, Hoffman J, Apfel R, et al. Effects of glatiramer acetate on fatigue and days of absence from work in first-time treated relapsing-remitting multiple sclerosis. Health Qual Life Outcomes 2008;6:67.

90. Metz LM, Patten SB, Archibald JC, et al. The effect of immunomodulatory treatment on multiple sclerosis fatigue. J Neurol Neurosurg Psychiatry 2004;75:1045–7.

91. Lebrun C, Alchaar H, Bourg V, et al. Levocarnitine administration in multiple sclerosis patients with immunosuppressive therapy-induced fatigue. Mult Scler 2006;12(3):321–4.

92. Strober LB, Arnett PA. An examination of four models predicting fatigue in multiple sclerosis. Arch Clin Neuropsychol 2005;20(5):631–46.

93. Stanton BR, Barnes F, Silber E. Sleep and fatigue in multiple sclerosis. Mult Scler 2006;12(4):481–6.

94. Attarian H, Brown K, Duntley S, et al. The relationship of sleep disturbances and fatigue in multiple sclerosis. Arch Neurol 2004;61:525–8.

95. Veauthier C, Radbruch H, Gaede G. Fatigue in multiple sclerosis is closely related to sleep disorders: a polysomnographic cross-sectional study. Mult Scler 2011;17(5):613–22.

96. Bohr KC, Haas J. Sleep related breathing disorders do not explain daytime fatigue in multiple sclerosis. Mult Scler 1998;4:289a.

97. Zifko U, Rupp M, Schwartz S, et al. Modafinil in treatment of fatigue in multiple sclerosis: results of an open-label study. J Neurol 2002;249(8):983–7.

98. Rammohan KW, Rosenberg JH, Lynn DJ, et al. Efficacy and safety of modafinil (Provigil®) for the treatment of fatigue in multiple sclerosis: a two centre phase 2 study. J Neurol Neurosurg Psychiatry 2002;72:179–83.

99. Stankoff B, Waubant E, Confavreux G, et al. Modafinil for fatigue in MS: a randomized placebo-controlled double-blind study. Neurology 2005;64(7):1139–43.

100. Cohen R, Fisher M. Amantadine treatment of fatigue associated with multiple sclerosis. Arch Neurol 1989;46(6):676–80.

101. Weinshenker BG, Penman M, Bass B, et al. A double-blind, randomized, crossover trial of pemoline in fatigue associated with multiple sclerosis. Neurology 1992;42(8):1468–71.

102. Brañas P, Jordan R, Fry-Smith A, et al. Treatments for fatigue in multiple sclerosis: a rapid and systematic review. Health Technol Assess 2000;4(27):1–61.

103. Geisler M, Sliwinski M, Coyle PK, et al. The effects of amantadine and pemoline on cognitive functioning in multiple sclerosis. Arch Neurol 1996;53(2):185–8.

104. Romberg A, Virtanen A, Ruutiainen J. Effects of a 6-month exercise program on patients with multiple sclerosis: a randomized study. Neurology 2004;63(11):2034–8.

105. Bjarnadottir OH, Konradsdottir AD, Reynisdottir K, et al. Multiple sclerosis and brief moderate exercise: a randomised study. Mult Scler 2007;13(6):776–82.

106. Motl RW, Gosney JL. Effect of exercise training on quality of life in multiple sclerosis: a meta-analysis. Mult Scler 2008;14(1):129–35.

107. van Kessel K, Moss-Morris R, Willoughby E, et al. A randomized controlled trial of cognitive behavior therapy for multiple sclerosis fatigue. Psychosom Med 2008;70(2):205–13.

108. Ghahari S, Leigh Packer T, Passmore AE. Effectiveness of an online fatigue self-management programme for people with chronic neurological conditions: a randomized controlled trial. Clin Rehabil 2010;24(8):727–44.

109. de Carvalho M, Motta R, Konrad G, et al. A randomized placebo-controlled cross-over study using a low frequency magnetic field in the treatment of fatigue in multiple sclerosis. Mult Scler 2012;18(1):82–9.

110. Vuletić V, Lezaić Z, Morović S. Post-stroke fatigue. Acta Clin Croat 2011;50(3):341–4.

111. Christensen D, Johnsen SP, Watt T, et al. Dimensions of post-stroke fatigue: a two-year follow-up study. Cerebrovasc Dis 2008;26:134–41.

112. Ingles J, Eskes G, Phillips S. Fatigue after stroke. Arch Phys Med Rehabil 1999;80(2):173–8.

113. Snaphaan L, van der Werf S, de Leeuw FE. Time course and risk factors of post-stroke fatigue: a prospective cohort study. Eur J Neurol 2011;18:611–7.

114. Andersen G, Christensen D, Kirkevold M, et al. Post-stroke fatigue and return to work: a 2-year follow-up. Acta Neurol Scand 2012;125:248–53.

115. Lynch J, Meade G, Grieg C, et al. Fatigue after stroke: the development and evaluation of a case definition. J Psychosom Res 2007;63(5):539–44.

116. Choi-Kwon S, Choi J, Kwon SU, et al. Fluoxetine is not effective in the treatment of poststroke fatigue: a double-blind, placebo-controlled study. Cerebrovasc Dis 2007;23:103–8.

117. McGeough E, Pollock A, Smith LN, et al. Interventions for post-stroke fatigue. Cochrane Database Syst Rev 2009;(3):CD007030.

118. Freidman J, Friedman H. Fatigue in Parkinson's disease. Neurology 1993;43(10):2016–8.

119. Karlsen K, Larsen JP, Tandberg E, et al. Fatigue in patients with Parkinson's disease. Mov Disord 1999;14:237–41.

120. Herlofson K, Larsen JP. The influence of fatigue on health-related quality of life in patients with Parkinson's disease. Acta Neurol Scand 2003;107:1–6.

121. Garber CE, Friedman J. Effects of fatigue on physical activity and function in patients with Parkinson's disease. Neurology 2003;60(7):1119–24.

122. Pavese N, Metta V, Bose S, et al. Fatigue in Parkinson's disease is linked to striatal and limbic serotonergic dysfunction. Brain 2010;133(1):3434–43.

123. Abe K, Takanashi M, Yanagihara T. Fatigue in patients with Parkinson's disease. Behav Neurol 2000;12(3):103–6.

124. Ziv I, Avraham M, Michealov Y, et al. Enhanced fatigue during motor performance in patients with Parkinson's disease. Neurology 1998;51(6):1583–6.

125. Chokroverty S, editor. Sleep disorders medicine: basic science, technical considerations and clinical aspects. 3rd edition. Philadelphia: Saunders-Elsevier; 2009.

126. Havlikova E, van Dijk JP, Rosenberger J, et al. Fatigue in Parkinson's disease is not related to excessive sleepiness or quality of sleep. J Neurol Sci 2008;270(1):107–13.

127. Lou JS, Kearns G, Benice T, et al. Levodopa improves physical fatigue in Parkinson's disease: a double-blind, placebo-controlled, crossover study. Mov Disord 2003;18(10):1108–14.

128. Dobkin RD, Allen L, Menza M. Cognitive-behavioral therapy for depression in Parkinson's disease: a pilot study. Mov Disord 2007;22(7):946–52.

129. Buchwald D, Umali P, Umali J, et al. Chronic fatigue and the chronic fatigue syndrome: prevalence in a Pacific Northwest health care system. Ann Intern Med 1995;123(2):81–8.

130. Wessely S, Chalder T, Hirsch S, et al. The prevalence and morbidity of chronic fatigue and chronic fatigue syndrome: a prospective primary care study. Am J Public Health 1997;87(9):1449–55.

131. Jason L, Richman J, Rademaker A, et al. A community-based study of chronic fatigue syndrome. Arch Intern Med 1999;159:2129–37.

132. Nater UM, Lin JM, Maloney EM, et al. Psychiatric comorbidity in persons with chronic fatigue syndrome identified from the Georgia population. Psychosom Med 2009;71(5):557–65.

133. Wessely S, Powell R. Fatigue syndromes: a comparison of chronic "postviral" fatigue with neuromuscular and affective disorders. J Neurol Neurosurg Psychiatry 1989;52:940–8.

134. Hickie I, Lloyd A, Wakefield D, et al. The psychiatric status of patients with the chronic fatigue syndrome. Br J Psychiatry 1990;156:534–40.

135. Fukuda K, Straus S, Hickie I, et al. The chronic fatigue syndrome: a comprehensive approach to its definition and study. Ann Intern Med 1994;121:953–9.

136. Buchwald D, Ashley RL, Pearlman T, et al. Viral serologies in patients with chronic fatigue and chronic fatigue syndrome. J Med Virol 1996;50:25–30.

137. Mawle A, Nisenbaum R, Dobbins J, et al. Seroepidemiology of chronic fatigue syndrome: a case-control study. Clin Infect Dis 1995;21(6):1386–9.

138. Lombardi VC, Ruscetti FW, Das Gupta J, et al. Detection of an infectious retrovirus, XMRV, in blood cells of patients with chronic fatigue syndrome. Science 2009;326:585–9.

139. Satterfield B, Garcia R, Jia H, et al. Serologic and PCR testing of persons with chronic fatigue syndrome in the United States shows no association with xenotropic or polytropic murine leukemia virus-related viruses. Retrovirology 2011;8:12.

140. Landay AL, Lennett ET, Jessop C. Chronic fatigue syndrome: clinical condition associated with immune activation. Lancet 1991;338(8769):707–12.

141. Lorussoa L, Mikhaylovab S, Capellic E, et al. Immunological aspects of chronic fatigue syndrome. Autoimmun Rev 2009;8(4):287–91.

142. Schillings ML, Kalkmanb JS, van der Werf SP, et al. Diminished central activation during maximal voluntary contraction in chronic fatigue syndrome. Clin Neurophysiol 2004;115:2518–24.

143. Mariman A, Vogelaers D, Hanoulle I, et al. Subjective sleep quality and daytime sleepiness in a large sample of patients with chronic fatigue syndrome (CFS). Acta Clin Belg 2012;67(1):19–24.

144. Morriss R, Sharpe M, Sharpley AL, et al. Abnormalities of sleep in patients with the chronic fatigue syndrome. BMJ 1993;306:1161.

145. Krupp L, Jandorf L, Coyle PK, et al. Sleep disturbance in chronic fatigue syndrome. J Psychosom Res 1993;37(4):325–31.

146. Buchwald D, Pascauly R, Bombardier C, et al. Sleep disorders in patients with chronic fatigue. Clin Infect Dis 1994;18(S1):S68–72.

147. Sharpley A, Clements A, Hawton K, et al. Do patients with "pure" chronic fatigue syndrome (neurasthenia) have abnormal sleep? Psychosom Med 1997;59(6):592–6.

148. Fischler B, Le Bon O, Hoffmann G, et al. Sleep anomalies in the chronic fatigue syndrome. Neuropsychobiology 1997;35:115–22.

149. Manu P, Lane T, Matthews D, et al. Alpha-delta sleep in patients with a chief complaint of chronic fatigue. South Med J 1994;87(4):465–70.

150. McKenzie R, O'Fallon A, Dale J, et al. Low-dose hydrocortisone for treatment of chronic fatigue syndrome: a randomized controlled trial. JAMA 1998; 280(12):1061–6.

151. Moorkens G, Wynants H, Abs R. Effect of growth hormone treatment in patients with chronic fatigue syndrome: a preliminary study. Growth Horm IGF Res 1998;8(Suppl 2):131–3.

152. Peterson P, Shepard J, Macres M, et al. A controlled trial of intravenous immunoglobulin G in chronic fatigue syndrome. Am J Med 1990;89(5):554–60.

153. Lloyd A, Hickie I, Wakefield D, et al. A double-blind, placebo-controlled trial of intravenous immunoglobulin therapy in patients with chronic fatigue syndrome. Am J Med 1990;89(5):561–8.

154. Vollmer-Conna U, Hickie I, Hadzi-Pavlovic D, et al. Intravenous immunoglobulin is ineffective in the treatment of patients with chronic fatigue syndrome. Am J Med 1997;103(1):38–43.

155. Deale A, Chalder T, Marks I. Cognitive behavior therapy for chronic fatigue syndrome: a randomized controlled trial. Am J Psychiatry 1997;154:408–14.

156. Malouff J, Thorsteinsson E, Rooke S. Efficacy of cognitive behavioral therapy for chronic fatigue syndrome: a meta-analysis. Clin Psychol Rev 2008;28(5):736–45.

157. Butler S, Chalder T, Ron M, et al. Cognitive behaviour therapy in chronic fatigue syndrome. J Neurol Neurosurg Psychiatry 1991;54(2):153–8.

158. Delae A, Chaldera T, Wesselya S. Illness beliefs and treatment outcome in chronic fatigue syndrome. J Psychosom Res 1998;45(1):77–83.

159. Prins J, Bleijenberg G, Bazelmans E, et al. Cognitive behaviour therapy for chronic fatigue syndrome: a multicentre randomised controlled trial. Lancet 2001;357(9259):841–847,.

160. Deale A, Husain K, Chalder T, et al. Long-term outcome of cognitive behavior therapy versus relaxation therapy for chronic fatigue syndrome: a 5-year follow-up study. Am J Psychiatry 2001;158:2038–42.

161. Freidberg F, Krupp L. A comparison of cognitive behavioral treatment for chronic fatigue syndrome and primary depression. Clin Infect Dis 1994; 18(Suppl 1):S105–10.

162. de Lange F, Koers A, Kalkman J. Increase in prefrontal cortical volume following cognitive behavioural therapy in patients with chronic fatigue syndrome. Brain 2008;131(8):2172–80.

163. Fulchera K, White P. Randomised controlled trial of graded exercise in patients with the chronic fatigue syndrome. BMJ 1997;314(7095):1647–52.

164. Powell P, Bentall R, Nye F. Randomised controlled trial of patient education to encourage graded exercise in chronic fatigue syndrome. BMJ 2001;322(7283):387.

165. Neill J, Belan I, Ried K. Effectiveness of non-pharmacological interventions for fatigue in adults with multiple sclerosis, rheumatoid arthritis, or systemic lupus erythematosus: a systematic review. J Adv Nurs 2006;56:617–35.

166. Cairns R, Hotopf M. A systematic review describing the prognosis of chronic fatigue syndrome. Occup Med (Lond) 2005;55(1):20–31.

167. Wearden AJ, Morriss RK, Strickland PL, et al. Randomised, double-blind, placebo-controlled treatment trial of fluoxetine and graded exercise for chronic fatigue syndrome. Br J Psychiatry 1998;172:485–90.

168. Vercoulen JH, Hoofs MP, Bleijenberg G, et al. Randomised, double-blind, placebo-controlled study of fluoxetine in chronic fatigue syndrome. Lancet 1996;347(9005):858–61.

169. Hill N, Tiersky L, Scavella V, et al. Natural history of severe chronic fatigue syndrome. Arch Phys Med Rehabil 1999;80(9):1090–4.

170. Joyce J, Hotopf M, Wessley S. The prognosis of chronic fatigue and chronic fatigue syndrome: a systematic review. QJM 1997;90(3):223–33.

171. Rimes K, Goodman R, Hotopf M, et al. Incidence, prognosis, and risk factors for fatigue and chronic fatigue syndrome in adolescents: a prospective community study. Pediatrics 2007; 119(3):e603–9.

172. Gill A, Dosen A, Ziegler J. Chronic fatigue syndrome in adolescents: a follow-up study. Arch Pediatr Adolesc Med 2004;158:225–9.

173. Mills PJ, Kim J, Bardwell W, et al. Predictors of fatigue in obstructive sleep apnea. Sleep Breath 2008;12(4):397–9.

174. Bardwell WA, Moore P, Anconi-Israel S, et al. Fatigue in obstructive sleep apnea: driven by depressive symptoms instead of apnea severity? Am J Psychiatry 2003;160:350–5.

175. Aguillard RN, Riedel BW, Lichstein KL, et al. Daytime functioning in obstructive sleep apnea patients: exercise tolerance, subjective fatigue, and sleepiness. Appl Psychophysiol Biofeedback 1998;23(4):207–17.

176. Yue HJ, Bardwell W, Ancoli-Israel S, et al. Arousal frequency is associated with increased fatigue in obstructive sleep apnea. Sleep Breath 2009;13: 331–9.

177. Tomfohr LM, Ancoli-Israel S, Loredo JS, et al. Effects of continuous positive airway pressure on fatigue and sleepiness in patients with obstructive sleep apnea: data from a randomized controlled trial. Sleep 2011;34(1):121–6.

178. Droogleever Fortuyn HA, Fronczek R, Smitshoek M, et al. Severe fatigue in narcolepsy with cataplexy. J Sleep Res 2012;21(2):163–9.

179. Becker PM, Schwartz JR, Feldman N, et al. Effect of modafinil on fatigue, mood, and health-related quality of life in patients with narcolepsy. Psychopharmacology 2004;171(2):133–9.

180. Cuellar NG, Ratcliffe SJ. A comparison of glycemic control, sleep, fatigue, and depression in type 2 diabetes with and without restless legs syndrome. J Clin Sleep Med 2008;4(1):50–6.

181. Oliveira AR, Correa FI, Correa JC, et al. Analysis of fatigue associated to periodic limb movement during sleep in former poliomyelitis patients. Rev Neurol 2012;54(1):24–30 [in Spanish].

Psychiatric Disorders and Fatigue

John Herman, PhD

KEYWORDS

- Depression • Insomnia • Obstructive sleep apnea • ADHD • Anxiety • Dementia • Sleepiness
- Buproprion

KEY POINTS

- Fatigue and psychiatric disorders often coexist.
- When the chief complaint is fatigue, a psychiatric disorder is 10 times more likely than chronic fatigue syndrome.
- Many patients with sleep disorders complain of fatigue.
- Patients with depressive disorders complain of chronic fatigue but frequently deny depression.
- Antidepressants with activating properties are effective in treating fatigue.

INTRODUCTION

Because obstructive sleep apnea disrupts sleep and causes multiple awakenings, some patients with obstructive sleep apnea report insomnia. However, it also causes daytime sleepiness, and many patients describe excessive sleepiness. This model is similar to how fatigue presents in psychiatric disorders. Some patients complain of depression, mood swings, anxiety, irritability, or panic attacks and seek therapy or medications for these symptoms. However, each of these symptoms is strongly associated with fatigue. Other patients with these symptoms complain of fatigue and seek treatment. This article describes sleepiness and fatigue commonly seen in psychiatric disorders.

COMORBIDITY BETWEEN FATIGUE AND PSYCHIATRIC DISORDERS

Fatigue and psychiatric disorders frequently coexist. In one study examining the comorbidity between chronic fatigue and psychiatric disorders,[1] 135 consecutive patients with 6 months or more of debilitating fatigue were extensively evaluated for psychiatric and medical disorders. Assessment included a history and physical examination; blood tests; sleep studies (when indicated); and a well-validated questionnaire. Six of the patients met criteria for chronic fatigue syndrome (CFS); 91 (67%) patients had clinically active psychiatric disorders; and four had medical disorders that were considered a major cause of their fatigue. Another prospective study of 100 consecutive patients complaining of chronic fatigue found that 66 patients had one or more psychiatric disorders that could explain their fatigue symptoms.[2] Approximately half of these met diagnostic criteria for depression. Among other psychiatric disorders present, somatization disorder and anxiety disorders were diagnosed frequently.

When I reviewed the *Diagnostic and Statistical Manual of Mental Disorders, Fourth Edition*, 1994 (DSM IV), I found 32 of the 267 diagnoses to include a symptom or symptoms related to fatigue. A list of these disorders and the diagnostic symptoms listed in DSM IV for each of these disorders that overlap with fatigue follows. These symptoms are italicized. In many of the disorders that include the symptom of hypersomnia, there is also an insomnia subtype that could have chronic fatigue but is not included.

1. Attention-deficit/hyperactivity disorder (ADHD): *problems with attention, sustaining attention, not listening, avoids tasks that require sustained mental effort, easily distracted, fidgets,*

University of Texas Southwestern Medical Center at Dallas, Dallas, Texas 75390-9182, USA
E-mail address: john.herman@childrens.com

Sleep Med Clin 8 (2013) 213–219
http://dx.doi.org/10.1016/j.jsmc.2013.02.002
1556-407X/13/$ – see front matter © 2013 Published by Elsevier Inc.

demonstrates impulsivity. Each of these symptoms of ADHD could easily be a symptom of fatigue, especially the attention deficit subtype. Individuals with ADHD are more likely to have one or more sleep disorders but no studies have examined the relationship of it to fatigue.

2. Delirium: *disturbance of consciousness (ie, reduced clarity of awareness of the environment) with reduced ability to focus, sustain, or shift attention*. The disturbance in consciousness with reduced attention can be secondary to a medical condition, induced by a substance or withdrawal from a substance, or of unknown cause. The overlap with symptoms of fatigue is considerable but this has never been studied.

3. Alzheimer dementia: *memory impairment, inability to learn new information or to recall previously learned information, depressed mood*. The gradual onset of mild cognitive impairment in early Alzheimer disease inducing problems with memory, learning, and attention, and depressed mood could easily be confused with fatigue. Fatigue might be seen as causing this symptom cluster. It is clinically difficult to distinguish mild cognitive impairment from chronic fatigue because of the overlap of symptoms. The factor that might be the most helpful in distinguishing fatigue from early Alzheimer disease is the lack of insight of the impaired individual with regards to decline of function. The Alzheimers Association lists "feeling weary of work, family and social obligations" as one of the 10 early symptoms of cognitive decline, consistent with the overlap with fatigue.

4. Vascular dementia: *memory impairment, inability to learn new information or to recall previously learned information, depressed mood*. Vascular dementia, formerly called multi-infarct dementia, may present with focal neurologic symptoms, difficulties in functioning, or behavioral disturbances, in addition to the previously mentioned symptoms. Chronic fatigue could be viewed as an explanation to an individual with these symptoms who has not been properly diagnosed.

5. Dementia caused by other general medical conditions: *memory impairment, inability to learn new information or to recall previously learned information, depressed mood*. The early stages of many medical conditions, such as heart disease or cancer, frequently are accompanied by mild cognitive impairment because of reduced cerebral blood flow. Individuals could well explain such symptoms as chronic fatigue.

6. Substance-induced persisting dementia: *memory impairment, inability to learn new information or to recall previously learned information, depressed mood, cognitive deficits that cause significant occupational functioning*.

7. Dementia caused by multiple etiologies: *memory impairment, inability to learn new information or to recall previously learned information, depressed mood, cognitive deficits that cause significant occupational functioning*.

8. Amnestic disorder: *memory impairment, inability to learn new information or to recall previously learned information, depressed mood, cognitive deficits that cause significant occupational functioning*.

9. Substance-induced persisting amnestic disorder: *memory impairment, inability to learn new information or to recall previously learned information, depressed mood, cognitive deficits that cause significant occupational functioning*.

10. Personality change caused by a general medical condition, apathetic type: *marked by apathy and indifference*.

11. Substance intoxication: *impaired occupational functioning*. Intoxication with and withdrawal from alcohol or drugs of abuse is characterized by a sense of fatigue, problems with memory, decision making, and learning new subject matter. Because information about substance abuse is not forthcoming, in most cases, the substance abuser is more likely to complain of chronic fatigue. This applies to the next seven DSM IV diagnoses.

12. Substance withdrawal: *impaired occupational functioning*.

13. Alcohol intoxication: *impaired attention or memory, impaired social or occupational functioning*.

14. Amphetamine withdrawal: *fatigue, psychomotor retardation*.

15. Cocaine withdrawal: *fatigue, hypersomnia, psychomotor retardation*.

16. Inhalant intoxication: *lethargy, psychomotor retardation, generalized muscle weakness*.

17. Opioid intoxication: *drowsiness, impaired attention or memory, apathy, psychomotor retardation*.

18. Sedative, hypnotic, or anxiolytic intoxication: *impaired social or occupational functioning, impaired attention or memory*.

19. Schizoaffective disorder, depressive type: meets criteria for major depressive disorder.

20. Major depressive disorder: *marked diminished interest or pleasure in activities, hypersomnia,*

nonrestorative sleep, psychomotor retardation, fatigue, inability to concentrate. This is the most frequent psychiatric diagnosis for individuals presenting with chronic fatigue. Patients complaining of chronic fatigue are far more likely to meet diagnostic criteria for major depressive disorder than CFS. Many individuals experience each and every one of their depressive symptoms as a fatigue symptom. Some abhor a psychiatric diagnosis and cling to their fatigue explanation. Some blame their fatigue on poor sleep, not recognizing nonrefreshing sleep as a symptom of depression. Although fatigue has no official definition, the terms used to describe it overlap with the description of major depressive disorder and dysthymic disorder sufficiently to cause confusion for many patients and physicians. This overlap is extensive enough to raise the question of a commonality of fatigue and depression for a subset of patients. Several recent studies have asserted that fatigue is inheritable, claiming that it runs in families.[3] These studies were not large enough to estimate a rate of heritability.

The assertion of heritability raises three questions. (1) Does chronic fatigue have a genetic component? (2) Might there be an overlap between genes involved in the heritability of depression and fatigue? (3) Are fatigue and depression, in some instances, different manifestations of a common disorder?

21. Dysthymic disorder: *hypersomnia, low energy or fatigue, poor concentration*. Similar to major depressive disorder, but less intense and more likely to be chronic, many individuals with dysthymia describe themselves as fatigued. Two of the descriptors of dysthymic disorder in DSM IV include fatigue and low energy.

22. Bipolar disorder, depressed episode: meets criteria for major depressive disorder with a history of a manic episode.

23. Bipolar disorder II, depressed episode: meets criteria for major depressive disorder with a history of a hypomanic episode.

24. Mood disorder caused by a general medical condition: *caused by physiologic effects of a general medical condition, diminished interest or pleasure, irritability, fatigue, hypersomnia, inability to concentrate*. Fatigue is an early symptom of many medical conditions, similar to depression. Before diagnosis of the underlying medical cause, many individuals describe chronic fatigue as the explanation for their decreased energy and other symptoms.

25. Substance-induced mood disorder with depressive features: meets criteria for dysthymic disorder.

26. Seasonal affective disorder: meets criteria for major depressive disorder or dysthymic disorder in conjunction with episodes beginning in fall or winter.

27. Posttraumatic stress disorder: *numbing of general responsiveness, diminished interest or participation in significant activities, restricted affect, difficulty falling or staying asleep, difficulty concentrating*. Posttraumatic stress disorder disrupts the hypothalamic-pituitary-adrenal axis, causing chronic secretion of stress hormones, impairing the ability of these hormones to be available in increased amounts during waking activities. This is associated with a sense of chronic fatigue and the symptoms listed previously.

28. Generalized anxiety disorder: *becoming easily fatigued; difficulty concentrating or mind goes blank; difficulty falling asleep, staying asleep, or nonrestorative sleep; impairment in occupational or social functioning*. Studies of individuals complaining of chronic fatigue show a fourfold increase in anxiety disorders compared with control subjects.[4] Individuals with chronic anxiety lose an energy reserve, instead becoming easily fatigued. Their impairment in social or occupational functioning is experienced as being caused by fatigue.

29. Primary insomnia: *daytime fatigue, nonrestorative sleep*. One of the identifying criteria of insomnia is disrupted sleep followed by the inability to nap when given the opportunity. Insomniacs typically complain of fatigue and have many symptoms overlapping with CFS.

30. Primary hypersomnia: *excessive sleepiness, daytime sleep episodes, nonrestorative sleep*. Primary hypersomnia or idiopathic hypersomnia is characterized by a normal or extended period of sleep followed by the sensation of lethargy or fatigue. It is of note that all of the insomnias and hypersomnias share in common daytime fatigue.

31. Circadian rhythm sleep disorder: *insomnia, excessive daytime sleepiness that causes significant distress or impairment in occupational or social functioning*. Individuals with delayed sleep phase disorder experience themselves as fatigued, sleepy, and lethargic in the morning. Individuals with advanced sleep phase disorder become fatigued and sleepy in the evening.

32. Sleep disorder caused by a general medical condition: *nonrestorative sleep, excessive daytime sleepiness, insomnia, hypersomnia*.

Several published studies confirm the high prevalence of psychiatric disorders being present in patients complaining of chronic fatigue with rates varying between 44% and 80%. Chronic fatigue is not considered a psychiatric disorder, although psychiatrists sometimes use the diagnosis of somatoform disorder NOS, which is not listed here because no words implying fatigue are used in defining this condition.

FATIGUE AND SLEEP DISORDERS

Sleep disorders also occur conjointly with psychiatric disorders and chronic fatigue. One prospective study examined the prevalence of sleep disorders in patients with chronic fatigue. A series of patients complaining of chronic fatigue were medically and psychiatrically evaluated and underwent a sleep study. Criteria for CFS were met by two-thirds of patients and those for a current psychiatric disorder were met by more than half of patients. Overall, almost half of the patients had abnormal results for a multiple sleep latency test and more than 80% had at least one sleep disorder, most frequently sleep apnea and idiopathic hypersomnia. Chronically fatigued patients may have potentially treatable coexisting sleep disorders and psychiatric disorders.

One study examined the relationship between obstructive sleep apnea, fatigue, and depression. The study determined that fatigue in patients with obstructive sleep apnea is best accounted for by their sleep-disordered breathing or by their depressive symptoms. The authors studied patients with severe obstructive sleep apnea who complained of fatigue. All patients were studied by polysomnogram and each completed a depression scale and a fatigue scale. They found that severity of obstructive sleep apnea on the sleep study only accounted for 4% of the variance in fatigue, but that the score on the depression scale accounted for almost half of the variance in fatigue. When obstructive sleep apnea severity was controlled, higher levels of depressive symptoms were strongly associated with greater levels of fatigue. These authors advocate treating the sleep-disordered breathing and the associated residual depression.[5]

DISTINGUISHING FATIGUE FROM SLEEPINESS

There is no laboratory test or biomarker for fatigue unlike the ability to measure sleepiness. Sleep studies, such as the Multiple Sleep Latency Test and the Maintenance of Wakefulness Test, can objectively measure sleepiness. Both fatigue and sleepiness are common to many illnesses.

Some tests of continuous performance objectively measure fatigue in normal subjects, but are not necessarily useful for evaluating individual patients.[6] For example, on a continuous performance test of simple addition problems, the subject's speed and accuracy deteriorate after a prolonged period of testing. If the individual takes a break, with or without sleep, when he or she returns to the addition test, performance improves. This is an objective measure of fatigue in a laboratory setting, but it has limited relevance to patients who complain of chronic fatigue.

During an evaluation, individuals are deemed sleepy if they state that they can easily fall asleep currently given a quiet and dark room with a bed. No matter what words an individual uses, such as tired, drained, sleepy, exhausted, or worn-out, fatigue is considered present if the individual states that he or she would not be able to fall asleep given a quiet and dark bedroom.

Part of the Centers for Disease Control and Prevention definition of CFS is helpful in distinguishing fatigue from sleepiness. The definition is widely accepted but has questionable sensitivity and specificity[7]:

1. Impaired memory or concentration
2. Postexertional malaise, where physical or mental exertions bring on "extreme, prolonged exhaustion and sickness"
3. Unrefreshing sleep
4. Muscle pain (myalgia)
5. Pain in multiple joints (arthralgia)
6. Headaches of a new kind or greater severity
7. Sore throat, frequent or recurring
8. Tender lymph nodes (cervical or axillary)

Diagnosing CFS by the Centers for Disease Control and Prevention definition requires that the patient endorse four of the eight items. Some of these are not symptomatic of a sleep disorder or sleepiness, especially postexertional malaise, muscle pain, pain in multiple joints, sore throat, and tender lymph nodes. However, impaired memory or concentration and unrefreshing sleep are also symptoms of insomnia. The inability to fall asleep when feeling tired or fatigued is common in insomnia, which is why five of the items listed previously are helpful for differentiating fatigue from a sleep disorder.

A medical or psychiatric work-up for fatigue versus sleepiness includes a history and physical. In performing an examination for fatigue, the approximate date of the onset of fatigue and its course over time should be thoroughly examined.

Medical causes, psychiatric disorders, and stressors should be evaluated.

After the examiner has determined that fatigue is present and has been present for 6 months, and a psychiatric diagnosis is established, the next step in the evaluation is to determine if a sleep disorder is possibly present. If a sleep disorder is likely present, begin the evaluation with a sleep study. A Maintenance of Wakefulness Test or Multiple Sleep Latency Test may be obtained if daytime sleepiness is likely.

PSYCHIATRIC EVALUATION OF THE PATIENT WITH CHRONIC FATIGUE

An in-depth interview of the patient with chronic fatigue includes questions about current stressors, occupational, marital, financial, and social concerns. One should pursue in detail the onset of the chronic fatigue and inquire about stressors that occurred at that time. Inquiry about head injury or concussions at any time is relevant.

Standardized and validated assessment scales are also useful. Some are brief enough for a patient to complete rapidly. The short form of the Profile of Mood States (POMS) is a 37-item questionnaire asking the patient to rate each item from zero to four, or not relevant to extremely relevant to their mood in the past 24 hours.[8] One rates such items as anger, sadness, nervousness, worthlessness, inability to concentrate, helplessness, and restlessness. Subscales of the POMS include tension-anxiety, anger-hostility, fatigue-inertia, vigor-activity, and confusion-bewilderment. The reliability and validity of the short form of the POMS has been established.[9]

If a psychiatric diagnosis is established for a patient with chronic fatigue, treating it with psychotropic medications or cognitive-behavioral therapy is a next step. The most frequent diagnosis emerging when a patient complains of chronic fatigue is depression, either major depressive disorder or dysthymia.

One of the most widely accepted and well validated brief scales for rating depression is the Hamilton Rating Scale for Depression.[10] This scale is to be administered by a health care professional. It evaluates depressed mood and suicidality, and 18 other symptoms linked to depression. The most commonly used brief instrument for rating anxiety is the Hamilton Anxiety Scale,[11] a 14-question scale administered by a health care provider. One of the most frequently used scales for evaluating sleep quality, insomnia, sleep disorders including obstructive sleep apnea, and daytime sleepiness is the Pittsburgh Sleep Quality Index.[12] The standard scale

for assessing daytime sleepiness is the Epworth Sleepiness Scale.[13] This is an eight-question, four-point, self-administered scale in which the individual judges if he or she would never doze or sleep under certain conditions, at one extreme, or has a high chance of dozing or sleeping at the other extreme. Each of these scales is available on the Internet.

TREATMENT OF THE INDIVIDUAL COMPLAINING OF CHRONIC FATIGUE THAT HAS A PSYCHIATRIC DIAGNOSIS

Using the previously mentioned interview techniques and questionnaires, a psychiatric diagnosis may be established that best explains the chronic fatigue symptoms. It is requisite that the health care provider establishing a psychiatric diagnosis rule out underlying medical conditions, as described in the review of DSM IV discussed previously in this article. Accurate diagnosis is just a first step in treating the complaint of chronic fatigue. Following the patient through successful amelioration of symptoms is requisite.

Frequently, patients complaining of fatigue are resistant to accept a psychiatric diagnosis. In such cases, it is best if the health care provider agree with the patient that fatigue is at the root of the problem and explain that the recommended psychotropic medication treats fatigue. After the patient begins a medication it is critical that the health care provider follow-up with the patient until it is determined if the selected medication is efficacious at alleviating the presenting symptoms. If not, it might be necessary to modify dosage or change medications. All psychotropics have multiple side effects and these should be monitored. In some cases, referral to a psychiatrist might be in the patient's best interest if there is treatment resistance or there is a lack of response to medications.

The following treatments are from an article published in the journal *Psychiatry* related to the Baltimore epidemiologic catchment area follow-up study.[14]

Cognitive Therapy

Cognitive behavioral therapy (CBT) is always an option for residual depression with fatigue.[15,16] The form of CBT used in residual fatigue is similar to the CBT used to treat somatoform disorders, CFS, and fibromyalgia.[17]

Graded Exercise

Besides improving physical condition, sustained exercise may improve mood itself. Exercise is used along with CBT in patients who complain of fatigue and depression and have no history of physical activity.[18] It is important to start gradually and increase intensity slowly.

Pharmacologic Interventions

There are practically no prospective studies addressing the specific effects of medications on residual fatigue. However, the experience in treatment-resistant depression with such medications as stimulants, thyroid preparations, and more recently with selegiline, modafinil, and armodafinil is considerable.

Bupropion's mechanism of action involves dopaminergic and noradrenergic receptors. It has an alerting effect and inhibits sleep. Even though there are no prospective studies in residual chronic fatigue after a patient has been treated with a selective serotonin reuptake inhibitor (SSRI), bupropion is likely a more effective drug in these patients.[19]

SSRIs as a group are not effective in the treatment of chronic fatigue. In general, SSRIs effectively treat depression but have a limited effect on fatigue. One-third of depressed patients who responded to fluoxetine had fatigue as a residual symptom. In a comparison with exercise in CFS, fluoxetine only improved depression, whereas graded exercise improved fatigue. A double-blind study did not show difference among fluoxetine, paroxetine, and sertraline regarding fatigue.[20]

Stimulants seem to improve fatigue in medical conditions, such as stroke, multiple sclerosis, cancer, HIV infection, and in elderly patients. D-amphetamine and methylphenidate have been shown to improve fatigue in patients with cancer.[21] Because these agents have abuse potential, patient selection is important.

Modafinil and armodafinil are approved for the treatment of narcolepsy, but are widely used to improve alertness in a variety of conditions. Studies have shown augmentation with modafinil in the treatment of fatigue in multiple sclerosis.[22] A relatively large placebo-controlled study of modafinil for fatigue in depression showed modafinil to be effective rapidly but to lose efficacy over time.[23]

A variety of agents approved for the treatment of Parkinson disease have shown efficacy in the treatment of chronic fatigue. These include amantadine,[24] pergolide,[25] and selegiline,[26] each of which increases vigor in chronic fatigue.

Thyroid levels, even in the normal range, might benefit from augmentation.[27] The use of L-thyroxine (0.5 mg) in euthyroid individuals improved depression and fatigue, especially in women.[28]

In selecting a treatment for a psychiatric patient with chronic fatigue, it should be tailored specifically to the psychiatric diagnosis. For example, anxiety disorders do not benefit from stimulants. Drug-induced chronic fatigue or drug withdrawal chronic fatigue makes the selection of a pharmacotherapy complex. CBT or graded exercise are indicated in many patients in whom pharmacotherapy is not indicated.

REFERENCES

1. Manu P, Lane TJ, Matthews DA. The frequency of the chronic fatigue syndrome in patients with symptoms of persistent fatigue. Ann Intern Med 1988; 109(7):554–6.
2. Buchwald D, Pearlman T, Kith W, et al. Screening for psychiatric disorders in chronic fatigue and chronic fatigue syndrome. J Psychosom Res 1997; 42(1):87–94.
3. Albright F, Light K, Light A, et al. Evidence for a heritable predisposition to chronic fatigue syndrome. BMC Neurol 2011;11:62. http://dx.doi.org/10.1186/1471-2377-11-62.
4. Donovan KA, Jacobsen PB. The Fatigue Symptom Inventory: a systematic review of its psychometric properties. Support Care Cancer 2010; 19(2):169–85.
5. Bardwell WA, Moore P, Ancoli-Israel S, et al. Fatigue in obstructive sleep apnea: driven by depressive symptoms instead of apnea severity? Am J Psychiatry 2003;160(2):350–5.
6. Dinges DI, Powell JW. Microcomputer analysis of performance on a portable, simple visual RT task sustained operations. Behav Res Meth Instrum Comput 1985;17:652–5.
7. Marin H, Menza MA. Specific treatment of residual fatigue in depressed patients. Psychiatry 2004; 1(2):12–8.
8. Pollock V, Cho DW, Reker D, et al. Profile of Mood States: the Factors and Their Physiological Correlates. The Journal of Nervous and Mental Disease 1979;167(10):612–4.
9. Yoshida K, Sekiguchi M, Otani K, et al. A validation study of the Brief Scale for Psychiatric problems in Orthopaedic Patients (BS-POP) for patients with chronic low back pain (verification of reliability, validity, and reproducibility). J Orthop Sci 2011; 16(1):7–13.
10. Hedlund JL, Vieweg BW. The Hamilton rating scale for depression. J Oper Psychiatr 1979;10(2):149–65.
11. Hamilton M. The assessment of anxiety states by rating. Br J Med Psychol 1959;32:50–5.
12. Buysee DJ, Reynolds F, Monk TH, et al. The Pittsburgh Sleep Quality Index: a new instrument for

psychiatric practice and research. Psychiatry Res 1989;28:183–213.

13. Johns MW. A new method for measuring daytime sleepiness: the Epworth sleepiness scale. Sleep 1991;14(6):540–5.

14. Marin H, Menza MA. Specific Treatment of Residual Fatigue in Depressed Patients. Psychiatry (Edgmont) 2004;1(2):12–8.

15. Fava GA, Grandy S, Zielezny M, et al. Cognitive behavioral treatment of residual symptoms in primary major depressive disorder. Am J Psychiatry 1994;151:1295–9.

16. Blackburn IM, Moore RG. Controlled acute and follow-up trial of cognitive therapy and pharmacotherapy in out-patients with recurrent depression. Br J Psychiatry 1997;171:328–34.

17. Allen LA, Woolfolk RL, Lehrer PM, et al. Cognitive behavioral therapy for somatization disorder: a preliminary investigation. J Behav Ther Exp Psychiatry 2001;32:53–62.

18. Powell P. Randomized controlled trial of patient education to encourage graded exercise in chronic fatigue syndrome. BMJ 2001;322:1–5.

19. Goodnick PJ, Sandoval R, Brickman A, et al. Bupropion treatment of fluoxetine-resistant chronic fatigue syndrome. Biol Psychiatry 1992;32:834–8.

20. Fava M, Hoog SL, Judge RA, et al. Acute efficacy of fluoxetine versus sertraline and paroxetine in major depressive disorder. J Clin Psychopharmacol 2002;22:137–47.

21. Olson LG, Ambrogetti A, Sutherland DC. A pilot randomized controlled trial of dexamphetamine in patients with chronic fatigue syndrome. Psychosomatics 2003;44:38–43.

22. Zifko UA, Rupp M, Schwarz S, et al. Modafinil in treatment of fatigue in multiple sclerosis: results of an open-label study. J Neurol 2002;249:983–7.

23. DeBattista C, Doghramji K, Menza MA, et al. Adjunct modafinil for the short-term treatment of fatigue and sleepiness in patients with major depressive disorder: a preliminary double-blind placebo controlled study. J Clin Psychiatry 2003; 64:1057–64.

24. Branas P, Jordan R, Fry-Smith A, et al. Treatments for fatigue in multiple sclerosis: a rapid and systematic review. Health Technol Assess 2000;4(27): 1–61.

25. Abe K, Takanashi M, Yanagihara T, et al. Pergolide mesylate may improve fatigue in patients with Parkinson's disease. Behav Neurol 2001–2002; 13(3–4):117–21.

26. Natelson BH, Cheu J, Hill N, et al. Single-blind, placebo phase-in trial of two escalating doses of selegiline in chronic fatigue syndrome. Neuropsychobiology 1998;37:150–9.

27. Andersen S, Pedersen KM, Bruun NH, et al. Narrow individual variations in serum T4 and T3 in normal subjects: a clue to the understanding of subclinical thyroid disease. J Clin Endocrinol Metab 2002;87: 1068–72.

28. Cox Dzurec L. Experiences of fatigue and depression before and after low-dose l-thyroxine supplementation in essentially euthyroid individuals. Res Nurs Health 1997;20:389–98.

Fatigue in Cardiorespiratory Conditions

Amir Sharafkhaneh, MD, PhD[a,b,*], Jose Melendez, MD[a],
Farah Akhtar, MD[a], Charlie Lan, DO[a]

KEYWORDS

- Congestive heart failure • Chronic obstructive pulmonary disease • Asthma • Sleep • Hypoxia

KEY POINTS

- Fatigue is frequently reported in patients with chronic cardiorespiratory conditions.
- Change in muscle structure and function, deteriorated nutritional status, sleep deprivation, hypoxia (awake, exertional and nocturnal), adverse effects of medications, and comorbid conditions are among many pathophysiologic mechanisms that may promote fatigue in patients.
- Comprehensive assessment of all the promoting causes is required for better understanding and management of fatigue in these patients.

INTRODUCTION

Fatigue is prevalent in chronic cardiorespiratory conditions. Fatigue is a symptom complex that affects the quality of life markedly. It correlates strongly with other measures of quality of life and depression. This article reviews fatigue and pathophysiologic mechanisms that promote fatigue in chronic cardiorespiratory conditions.

Definition

Despite being one of the most common symptoms of illness, affecting the acutely ill to those with chronic conditions such as cancer or end-stage renal disease, fatigue remains ambiguously defined. Ream and Richardson,[1] in their concept analysis of fatigue, discuss how, regardless of it being used as both a noun and a verb, the definition of fatigue shared these similar characteristics: fatigue follows exertion; it is associated with physical or mental weariness and exhaustion; it comprises comfortless, troublesome, or odious feelings (hence so-called fatigues are a punishment); and

fatigue causes decreased functional ability, which is often temporary. They also found 4 recurrent attributes when reviewing nursing and medical literature, defining fatigue as: (1) a total body feeling and experience, encompassing physical, cognitive and emotional dimensions; (2) an odious and unpleasant experience that causes distress, (3) a chronic and unrelenting phenomenon, and (4) a subjective experience dependent on an individual's perceptions.

In this concept analysis, there are 2 factors necessary for fatigue to occur in a medical context. First, a pathologic physical or psychological condition must exist. Second, individuals must have the capability to consciously and cognitively subjectively evaluate their feelings.

The consequences of fatigue on both physical and mental abilities are reflected in a person's routine functioning. Everyday activities are affected, including work, household chores, and self-care actions such as bathing and dressing. Fatigue can also manifest in behavioral and cognitive responses, causing irritability, impaired

This work is supported by the Department of Veterans Affairs Research and Development Care Line.
[a] Section of Pulmonary and Critical Care and Sleep Medicine, Baylor College of Medicine, 1 Baylor Plaza, Houston, TX 77030, USA; [b] Sleep Disorders and Research Center, Michael E. DeBakey VA Medical Center, 2002 Holcombe Boulevard, Houston, TX 77030, USA
* Corresponding author. Baylor College of Medicine, MEDVA Medical Center Building 100 (111i), Houston, TX 77030.
E-mail address: amirs@bcm.edu

concentration, poor decision making, forgetfulness, and lack of motivation. All of these factors affect overall quality of life.[1]

From pathophysiologic standpoint, a combination of factors promotes fatigue in cardiorespiratory conditions. Chronic cardiovascular or respiratory conditions result in changes in skeletal muscles. Poor nutrition and catabolic states seen in chronic cardiorespiratory conditions add to the problem. Continuing inflammation is proposed as one of the mechanisms that may cause fatigue. In addition, associated hypoxia adds to the problem. Disturbed sleep caused by insomnia or sleep-disordered breathing also complicates the situation. In addition, there are the adverse effects of medications that can promote fatigue.

CARDIAC DISEASES AND FATIGUE

Heart failure remains the most common cause of hospitalization and morbidity-mortality in the elderly population.[2] Its associated symptoms of dyspnea, lower extremity edema, and fatigue often prove debilitating to those affected. Although these symptoms may cause functional limitations, they also significantly affect patients' psychological and social welfare. Fatigue, as a frequent manifestation of heart failure, remains particularly hard to characterize, given its subjectivity and unquantifiable nature. However, it is important to effectively evaluate fatigue as a symptom because it has important and independent long-term prognostic implications.[3] It manifests physically, cognitively, and emotionally and physicians therefore need to identify it.[2]

Prognostic Implications

The importance of defining, recognizing, and targeting fatigue given its impact on prognosis in cardiac disease was shown in an analysis of the 3029 patients randomized in the Carvedilol or Metoprolol European Trial (COMET).[3] The aim of the study was to evaluate the relative importance of self-reported severity of symptoms as predictors of outcomes in congestive heart failure (CHF). Although the New York Heart Association classification as an indicator of functional status is used as a prognostic factor in CHF, the significance of fatigue as a factor was unknown. COMET was a multicenter, randomized (1:1), double-blind, parallel-group trial comparing the effect of carvedilol with metoprolol tartrate on morbidity and mortality in patients with CHF over a mean follow-up of 58 months. Symptoms of fatigue, breathlessness, and angina were quantified using a 5-point scale: (1) asymptomatic, (2) walking up stairs at a normal pace, (3) walking at a normal pace on a flat surface, (4) walking slowly on a flat surface or during washing or dressing, and (5) at rest. Patients also used a 5-point scale with very good and very poor at either extreme to rate their well-being. Patients had these assessments at baseline and then at 4-month intervals.

In a univariate analysis, fatigue was significantly related to reduced survival (P<.001) and the development of worsening heart failure. In a multivariate Cox regression analysis including the 16 baseline covariates (including demographics, New York Heart severity classification, baseline comorbid conditions, and baseline cardiovascular medications), fatigue still proved to be a significant predictor for worsening heart failure (relative risk 1.09 per unit; 95% confidence interval 1.02–1.17; $P = .02$). Multivariate regression analysis showed that fatigue offered an increased relative risk of 11% for mortality ($P = .009$), 26% for all-cause hospitalization (P<.0001), and 28% for worsening heart failure (P<.0001). These data show the importance of fatigue as a symptom given that its severity predicts an increased risk of death and morbidity. It is also a simple, low-cost factor in the overall evaluation of patients with heart failure that includes laboratory tests, radiographic information, and physical examination findings.

Evaluation of Fatigue

The literature review by Fini and de Almeida Lopes Monteiro da Cruz[2] showed the wide array of assessment tools used to characterize fatigue in people with heart failure. Quantitative means were most often used. Research studies ranged from those containing no description of how fatigue was assessed, to studies using an author-derived scale, and others that provided plain descriptions of patient reports. Some studies measured fatigue in terms of intensity, whereas others by its presence or absence. Because of this variety in assessment methods, it is difficult to integrate multiple results regarding the incidence and characteristics of fatigue. Despite this hindrance, the included studies showed a high frequency of fatigue in heart failure with a range of 69% to 88%, making it one of the most frequently reported symptoms.

It is important to differentiate clinically between the subjective perception of fatigue and the objective reduction in muscle strength with activity.[4] Three major types of exercise tests are used in practice: the symptom-limited progressive exercise test carried to the point of exhaustion; the test of endurance at a predetermined level of exercise (which is submaximal); and tests of submaximal exercise performance, such as the time taken to complete a typical walking task or the distance covered at a comfortable walking speed along a corridor (the corridor walking test) or a self-propelled treadmill.[4] The most common clinical measure of fatigue is the Borg scale, which can be graded separately for fatigue and dyspnea. Although fatigue remains a major complaint of patients, it is rare in practice to monitor this symptom or its progression.[4]

Causes of Fatigue in Heart Failure

Research regarding the causes of fatigue in cardiac disease has focused on vasoconstriction and endothelial dysfunction leading to impaired muscular blood flow.[4] Even with adequate blood flow, muscles can become fatigued if they have primary structural or functional abnormalities. Multiple causes of fatigue in heart failure have been postulated, including reduced cardiac output, reduced oxygen delivery, impaired muscle blood flow, and abnormal skeletal muscle.

In most of those with well-compensated chronic heart failure, cardiac output remains normal during the early periods of exercise but muscle blood flow is reduced. This reduction occurs as blood is diverted away from the muscles and there is a reduction in muscle size and its vascular bed.[5] This leads to muscular fatigue, although it is not clear which factor is the most causative. Increasing muscle blood flow by increasing cardiac output during exercise has not been shown to reduce fatigue,[6] possibly because the cardiac output was not the variable leading to acute muscle fatigue, or because the increased cardiac output was just passing through the skin circulation and not necessarily leading to increased muscle perfusion.

There are multiple means by which to enhance oxygen delivery to the body, including increasing hemoglobin content, and thereby the blood's oxygen-carrying capacity, or by supplementing inhaled oxygen during maximal exercise testing.[7] However, it remains unclear whether or not augmented oxygen delivery improves muscle fatigue.

During exercise, muscular blood flow is enhanced by increased arterial blood pressure, leading to increased cardiac output, and by dilation of arterioles in exercising skeletal muscle.[4] However, in the exercising patient with chronic heart failure, excess sympathetically mediated vasoconstriction, activation of the plasma renin-angiotensin system, and increased levels of endothelin all lead to impaired arteriolar vasodilation, which, in turn, leads to dampened muscular blood flow. Although angiotensin-converting enzyme (ACE) inhibitors do not acutely restore these vasodilatory effects, chronic ACE inhibitor therapy has been shown to increase femoral blood flow during exercise along with improved peak oxygen consumption.[4]

Even if cardiac output, oxygen delivery, and muscular blood flow were enhanced, these factors may not contribute to reductions in fatigue, suggesting intrinsic abnormalities of the skeletal muscle preventing them from using oxygen.[4] Two postulated causes of this include loss of muscle bulk or intrinsic metabolic defects. Muscle biopsies from patients with heart failure showed moderate atrophy and biochemical alterations.[8,9]

Associated Symptoms

There are many symptoms that have been reported in association with fatigue. The main symptom associated with fatigue is dyspnea. Dyspnea is also associated with sleep disorders and depression. A study comparing fatigue and other variables between those with heart failure and those without showed associations between fatigue, anxiety, and depression, independently of the sample, and that the three partially explained dyspnea variability in the heart failure sample.[10] Another factor correlated with fatigue in research was the body mass index: when higher than or equal to 25, fatigue was more intense.[11]

Insomnia and Fatigue

There are many risk factors associated with insomnia, including aging, sleep apnea, depression, and chronic medical illnesses such as CHF.[12] One review found that sleep-disordered breathing and insomnia were the most common causes of sleep disturbances in CHF. Insomnia occurred in 33% of all patients with CHF. The more frequently reported symptoms were inability to sleep in the supine position (51%), restless sleep (44%), trouble falling asleep (40%), and early awakening (39%). There was no correlation between these sleep complaints and the severity of their CHF or clinical status. Using the Epworth Sleepiness Scale (ESS), approximately 20% of participants in the Cardiovascular Health Study (total of 4578 elderly participants) were identified as being usually sleepy in the daytime.

The symptoms of heart failure (eg, pain, dyspnea, anxiety) clearly contribute to sleeplessness; however, the treatment regimens for this illness may also be playing a role. Current guidelines recommend multiple medications, including β-blockers, loop diuretics, ACE inhibitors, angiotensin II blockers, and aldosterone receptor blockers. Although these medications have been shown to improve morbidity and mortality from CHF, they may also be hindering sleep. In a study by Arzt and colleagues,[13] investigators reported sleep study and daytime sleepiness data from 155 optimally treated patients with CHF compared with 1139 controls from the same community. Patients with CHF compared with those without CHF, as measured by the ESS, had less subjective sleepiness. However, they did take longer to fall asleep, slept an average of an hour less per night, spent more time awake after falling asleep, had less rapid eye movement (REM) sleep and less deep non-REM sleep than did those without heart failure. In correlation with this study, in a questionnaire-based study of medication side effects in a hypertension clinic, lack of energy was the only symptom more prevalent in the treated than in the untreated. Although patients with CHF have worse sleep than those without CHF, it is not clear that they have more daytime sleepiness or that medications are the culprit.

There are not many data regarding sleep disturbances in CHF, given the under-recognition of the problem. This condition may be under-recognized partially because these patients tend to have less reported daytime sleepiness compared with patients without CHF. Because of lack of data, it is hard to say whether or not, or how much, medication to treat heart failure may be contributing to sleep irregularities. It is important for physicians to elicit symptoms from their patients regarding sleep symptoms given that addressing these issues may relieve secondary fatigue. There are no randomized trials evaluating insomnia in patients with heart failure, and clinical trials are necessary to ascertain what management strategies for insomnia in CHF may be effective.

RESPIRATORY DISORDERS AND FATIGUE

As in cardiac disease, patients with chronic obstructive pulmonary disease (COPD), interstitial lung disease (ILD), and other chronic respiratory conditions often present with fatigue as one of the main symptoms. COPD is the most studied of all the chronic respiratory conditions. In patients with COPD, fatigue is a common complaint from patients evaluated on a daily basis, being present in 68% to 80% of patients.[14–17] Similar to COPD, fatigue is also commonly reported in ILD. Assessment for the presence of fatigue is an integral part of the assessment of quality of life in lung diseases.[18] Fatigue out of proportion to lung function impairment may be considered a reason against lung transplantation and a reason for lung transplant evaluation in the case of a correlation with decline in lung function.[18,19] Fatigue is also

reported in other chronic respiratory conditions including cystic fibrosis and asthma.[20–22]

The pathophysiology of fatigue in COPD and ILD is not clear. Fatigue may result from the disease processes or adverse effects of the medications used. In chronic respiratory conditions, fatigue manifests as muscle weakness, poor exercise tolerance, and decrease in overall function. Chronic medical conditions including respiratory conditions result in a catabolic state and muscle breakdown and muscle atrophy that may manifest as fatigue.[23,24] Further, overlap between chronic respiratory conditions including COPD and sleep-related breathing disorders and insomnia can cause or intensify fatigue.[25,26]

In addition to the disease processes, use of various medications can promote fatigue. A classic example is chronic corticosteroid use in COPD for treatment of acute exacerbations or, in some rare instances, as a maintenance therapy. It is well known that steroids cause muscle fatigue and osteoporosis.[27,28] Some of respiratory inhalational medications can cause insomnia that may further promote fatigue.[26]

COPD

Various studies reported a high prevalence of chronic fatigue in patients with COPD (39%–58%).[29–31] In a survey comparing patients with COPD with the general population, Theander and colleagues[32] reported higher odds on frequency, duration, and severity of fatigue in patients with COPD. Further, 51% of patients with COPD reported fatigue as the worst or one of the worst symptoms.[32] Using Fatigue Impact Scale scores, patients with COPD reported higher scores in cognitive, physical, and psychological domains, indicating a significant effect on fatigue of this domain.[30]

Baltzan and colleagues[31] studied exercise capacity in patients with COPD with and without high fatigue scores. The group with high fatigue scores had lower exercise capacity, worse quality of life, worse depressive symptoms, and was less engaged in moderate-intensity activities. In a large study of 3000 patients with and without COPD, high fatigue score (using the Functional Assessment of Chronic Illness Therapy-Fatigue questionnaire) correlated with high depressive symptoms.[33,34] Baghai-Ravary and colleagues[35] studied 107 patients with COPD and 30 age-matched controls. The study showed that the increase in fatigue was associated with reduced time spent outdoors, depression, and exacerbation frequency. Further, fatigue increased during exacerbation episodes and this change was related to increased depression.[35]

Pathophysiology of fatigue in COPD is multifactorial. The work of breathing increases in COPD, resulting in increased resting metabolic demand up to twice the normal level.[14,15] The increased work of breathing is further complicated with altered nutrition, leading to muscle wasting and fatigue. Further, patients with advanced COPD may not be able to maintain adequate dietary intake (quantity and quality of nutrition) because of decreased appetite and physical and/or financial limitations. In turn, this results in cachexia and leads to weakness of the diaphragm and accessory muscles of ventilation, and creates a vicious cycle. Data indicate higher mortality in patients with COPD with lower body mass index.[36]

In addition to COPD-related pathophysiologic disturbances, presence of comorbid conditions, and particularly sleep deprivation, may promote fatigue in patient with COPD. Studies report a high prevalence of insomnia in patients with COPD.[26,37–39] The increased insomnia stems from COPD-related nocturnal symptoms and medication-related side effects that may disturb sleep.[26] In addition to insomnia, the presence of sleep-disordered breathing with COPD may increase fatigue.[25,26,40]

ILD

Fatigue and intolerance to physical activity are among early symptoms of ILD. The pathophysiologic mechanisms of fatigue related to ILD are muscle wasting, medications, depression, and factors associated with primary diseases like collagen vascular diseases. Presence of hypoxia; sleep disturbances, including insomnia; and other comorbid condition like heart failure further promotes fatigue in patients with ILD. In contrast with COPD, the progression of the ILD is unpredictable. The management of fatigue is important for the outcomes of patients with ILD, especially for patients who undergo lung transplantation.[41]

Unlike in COPD, the increased work of breathing in ILD is not caused by the loss of elasticity and subsequent active exhalation but rather by the loss of compliance of the lungs. In a systematic review of literature on quality of life in ILD, fatigue correlated strongly and significantly with dyspnea but not with lung function.[42] Sleep architecture, breathing mechanics, and oxygenation are affected adversely in patients with ILD.[43] High fatigue scores correlate with indices of low oxygen saturations during sleep.[44]

Fatigue is commonly reported in patients with sarcoidosis. Drent and colleagues[45] reported a fatigue prevalence of 66% in their cohort of patients with sarcoidosis. Female and young patients with sarcoidosis are affected more by fatigue.[46] Fatigue may present in the forms of early morning, intermittent, afternoon, or chronic fatigue.[47] Various factors, including the initial and residual inflammation and inflammatory profile (less competent Th2), are considered as the pathophysiologic mechanisms of fatigue in sarcoidosis.[47,48]

SUMMARY

Fatigue is frequently reported in patients with various chronic cardiorespiratory conditions. Change in muscle structure and function, deteriorated nutritional status, sleep deprivation, hypoxia (awake, exertional, and nocturnal), adverse effects of medications, and comorbid conditions are among many pathophysiologic mechanisms that may promote fatigue in patients. Comprehensive assessment of all the promoting causes is required for better understanding and management of fatigue in these patients.

REFERENCES

1. Ream E, Richardson A. Fatigue: a concept analysis. Int J Nurs Stud 1996;33:519–29.
2. Fini A, de Almeida Lopes Monteiro da Cruz D. Characteristics of fatigue in heart failure patients: a literature review. Rev Lat Am Enfermagem 2009;17:557–65.
3. Ekman I, Cleland JG, Swedberg K, et al. Symptoms in patients with heart failure are prognostic predictors: insights from COMET. J Card Fail 2005;11:288–92.
4. Drexler H, Coats AJ. Explaining fatigue in congestive heart failure. Annu Rev Med 1996;47:241–56.
5. Wilson JR, Martin JL, Schwartz D, et al. Exercise intolerance in patients with chronic heart failure: role of impaired nutritive flow to skeletal muscle. Circulation 1984;69:1079–87.
6. Mancini DM, Schwartz M, Ferraro N, et al. Effect of dobutamine on skeletal muscle metabolism in patients with congestive heart failure. Am J Cardiol 1990;65:1121–6.
7. Herrlin B, Nyquist O, Sylven C. Induction of a reduction in haemoglobin concentration by enalapril in stable, moderate heart failure: a double blind study. Br Heart J 1991;66:199–205.
8. Mancini DM, Walter G, Reichek N, et al. Contribution of skeletal muscle atrophy to exercise intolerance and altered muscle metabolism in heart failure. Circulation 1992;85:1364–73.
9. Lipkin DP, Jones DA, Round JM, et al. Abnormalities of skeletal muscle in patients with chronic heart failure. Int J Cardiol 1988;18:187–95.
10. Redeker NS. Somatic symptoms explain differences in psychological distress in heart failure patients vs a

comparison group. Prog Cardiovasc Nurs 2006;21: 182–9.

11. Tiesinga LJ, Dassen TW, Halfens RJ. DUFS and DEFS: development, reliability and validity of the Dutch Fatigue Scale and the Dutch Exertion Fatigue Scale. Int J Nurs Stud 1998;35:115–23.

12. Hayes D Jr, Anstead MI, Ho J, et al. Insomnia and chronic heart failure. Heart Fail Rev 2009;14:171–82.

13. Arzt M, Young T, Finn L, et al. Sleepiness and sleep in patients with both systolic heart failure and obstructive sleep apnea. Arch Intern Med 2006;166:1716–22.

14. Bartels MN. Fatigue in cardiopulmonary disease. Phys Med Rehabil Clin N Am 2009;20:389–404.

15. Celli BR, Cote CG, Marin JM, et al. The body-mass index, airflow obstruction, dyspnea, and exercise capacity index in chronic obstructive pulmonary disease 1. N Engl J Med 2004;350:1005–12.

16. Oga T, Nishimura K, Tsukino M, et al. Analysis of the factors related to mortality in chronic obstructive pulmonary disease: role of exercise capacity and health status. Am J Respir Crit Care Med 2003; 167:544–9.

17. McGavin CR, Gupta SP, Lloyd EL, et al. Physical rehabilitation for the chronic bronchitic: results of a controlled trial of exercises in the home. Thorax 1977;32:307–11.

18. Geertsma A, van der BW, de Boer WJ, et al. Survival with and without lung transplantation. Transplant Proc 1997;29:630–1.

19. Martinez FJ, Chang A. Surgical therapy for chronic obstructive pulmonary disease. Semin Respir Crit Care Med 2005;26:167–91.

20. Jarad NA, Sequeiros IM, Patel P, et al. Fatigue in cystic fibrosis: a novel prospective study investigating subjective and objective factors associated with fatigue. Chron Respir Dis 2012;9:241–9.

21. Brooks CM, Richards JM Jr, Bailey WC, et al. Subjective symptomatology of asthma in an outpatient population. Psychosom Med 1989;51:102–8.

22. Small SP, Lamb M. Measurement of fatigue in chronic obstructive pulmonary disease and in asthma. Int J Nurs Stud 2000;37:127–33.

23. Gosselink R, Troosters T, Decramer M. Peripheral muscle weakness contributes to exercise limitation in COPD. Am J Respir Crit Care Med 1996;153:976–80.

24. Mahler DA, Harver A. A factor analysis of dyspnea ratings, respiratory muscle strength, and lung function in patients with chronic obstructive pulmonary disease. Am Rev Respir Dis 1992;145:467–70.

25. Guilleminault C, Cummiskey J, Motta J. Chronic obstructive airflow disease and sleep studies. Am Rev Respir Dis 1980;122:397–406.

26. Sharafkhaneh A, Jayaraman G, Kaleekal T, et al. Sleep disorders and their management in patients with COPD. Ther Adv Respir Dis 2009;3:309–18.

27. Davies L, Angus RM, Calverley PM. Oral corticosteroids in patients admitted to hospital with exacerbations of chronic obstructive pulmonary disease: a prospective randomised controlled trial. Lancet 1999;354:456–60.

28. Rich A. Corticosteroids and chronic obstructive pulmonary disease in the nursing home. J Am Med Dir Assoc 2005;6:S68–74.

29. Gift AG, Shepard CE. Fatigue and other symptoms in patients with chronic obstructive pulmonary disease: do women and men differ? J Obstet Gynecol Neonatal Nurs 1999;28:201–8.

30. Theander K, Unosson M. Fatigue in patients with chronic obstructive pulmonary disease. J Adv Nurs 2004;45:172–7.

31. Baltzan MA, Scott AS, Wolkove N, et al. Fatigue in COPD: prevalence and effect on outcomes in pulmonary rehabilitation. Chron Respir Dis 2011;8: 119–28.

32. Theander K, Jakobsson P, Torstensson O, et al. Severity of fatigue is related to functional limitation and health in patients with chronic obstructive pulmonary disease. Int J Nurs Pract 2008;14:455–62.

33. Al-shair K, Muellerova H, Yorke J, et al. Examining fatigue in COPD: development, validity and reliability of a modified version of FACIT-F scale. Health Qual Life Outcomes 2012;10:100.

34. Hanania NA, Mullerova H, Locantore NW, et al. Determinants of depression in the ECLIPSE chronic obstructive pulmonary disease cohort. Am J Respir Crit Care Med 2011;183:604–11.

35. Baghai-Ravary R, Quint JK, Goldring JJ, et al. Determinants and impact of fatigue in patients with chronic obstructive pulmonary disease. Respir Med 2009;103:216–23.

36. Landbo C, Prescott E, Lange P, et al. Prognostic value of nutritional status in chronic obstructive pulmonary disease. Am J Respir Crit Care Med 1999; 160:1856–61.

37. Flenley DC. Sleep in chronic obstructive lung disease. Clin Chest Med 1985;6:651–61.

38. George CF, Bayliff CD. Management of insomnia in patients with chronic obstructive pulmonary disease. Drugs 2003;63:379–87.

39. Klink M, Quan SF. Prevalence of reported sleep disturbances in a general adult population and their relationship to obstructive airways diseases. Chest 1987;91:540–6.

40. Chaouat A, Weitzenblum E, Krieger J, et al. Association of chronic obstructive pulmonary disease and sleep apnea syndrome. Am J Respir Crit Care Med 1995;151:82–6.

41. Sulica R, Teirstein A, Padilla ML. Lung transplantation in interstitial lung disease. Curr Opin Pulm Med 2001;7:314–22.

42. Swigris JJ, Kuschner WG, Jacobs SS, et al. Health-related quality of life in patients with idiopathic pulmonary fibrosis: a systematic review. Thorax 2005; 60:588–94.

43. Agarwal S, Richardson B, Krishnan V, et al. Interstitial lung disease and sleep: what is known? Sleep Med 2009;10:947–51.

44. Mermigkis C, Stagaki E, Amfilochiou A, et al. Sleep quality and associated daytime consequences in patients with idiopathic pulmonary fibrosis. Med Princ Pract 2009;18:10–5.

45. Drent M, Wirnsberger RM, de Vries J, et al. Association of fatigue with an acute phase response in sarcoidosis. Eur Respir J 1999;13:718–22.

46. Hinz A, Fleischer M, Brahler E, et al. Fatigue in patients with sarcoidosis, compared with the general population. Gen Hosp Psychiatry 2011;33:462–8.

47. Sharma OP. Fatigue in sarcoidosis: incompletely understood, inadequately treated. Curr Opin Pulm Med 2012;18:470–1.

48. Korenromp IH, Grutters JC, van den Bosch JM, et al. Reduced Th2 cytokine production by sarcoidosis patients in clinical remission with chronic fatigue. Brain Behav Immun 2011;25:1498–502.

Cancer-Related Fatigue and Sleep Disorders

Diwakar D. Balachandran, MD*, Saadia Faiz, MD,
Lara Bashoura, MD, Ellen Manzullo, MD

KEYWORDS

- Cancer-related fatigue • Sleep disorders • Sleep disturbance • Management

KEY POINTS

- Cancer-related fatigue (CRF) continues to be a major concern of patients and providers of cancer care.
- The symptoms are debilitating and can persist for many years after the cancer diagnosis and therapy.
- Further research is required to address the mechanisms of illness, including a better understanding of the complex interplay between the sleep system, circadian rhythms, inflammation, and the hypothalamic-pituitary axis.
- Genetic analysis and genomic studies need to be done to better understand which patients may be prone to CRF and which therapies may exacerbate these symptoms.
- Attention must be focused on understanding which comorbidities, including mood disturbance, sleep disturbance deconditioning, cardiovascular, and endocrine function, contribute to CRF.

One of the most frequent and disturbing complaints of patients with cancer is fatigue. Cancer-related fatigue (CRF) is defined subjectively in a National Comprehensive Cancer Network Clinical Practice Guideline as a distressing, persistent, and subjective sense of physical, emotional, and/or cognitive tiredness or exhaustion related to cancer or cancer treatment that is not proportional to recent activity and interferes with usual functioning.[1] The symptom of CRF is experienced by 70% to 100% of patients with cancer. In patients with metastatic disease, the prevalence of CRF exceeds 75%. Numerous clinical characteristics have been associated with CRF, including generalized weakness, mood disturbance, diminished mental concentration, insomnia or hypersomnia, and sleep disturbance. Decrements of physical, social, and cognitive functioning; treatment noncompliance; and emotional distress for both patients and their family members have been described as consequences of CRF. The clinical criteria for the diagnosis of CRF have been established by Cella and others[2] in the *International Classification of Disease, Tenth Revision* criteria for CRF. These criteria include having 6 or more of 11 symptoms that are chronically related to cancer or cancer therapy which causes functional impairment and are not thought to be related to a comorbid psychiatric disorder.[2]

MEASUREMENT OF CRF

Fatigue in patients with cancer has been underreported, underdiagnosed, and undertreated. One reason for the underdiagnoses is the lack of objective measures to evaluate fatigue. Self-reported measures have been the mainstay of measuring the subjective symptoms and severity of fatigue. A variety of such instruments exist. The Functional Assessment for Cancer Therapy-Fatigue is a 13-item scale that is able to detect clinically meaningful differences in fatigue scores in response to treatment.[3] Another widely used multidimensional scale is the Fatigue Questionnaire.[4] This scale has

Department of Pulmonary Medicine, UT MD Anderson Cancer Center, Houston, Texas
* Corresponding author. Department of Pulmonary Medicine, UT MD Anderson Cancer Center, 1400 Pressler Street, Unit 1462, Houston, Texas 77030-4009, USA.
E-mail address: dbalachandran@mdanderson.org

Sleep Med Clin 8 (2013) 229–234
http://dx.doi.org/10.1016/j.jsmc.2013.02.005
1556-407X/13/$ – see front matter © 2013 Elsevier Inc. All rights reserved.

11 items that deal with both the physical and mental aspect of fatigue and was originally designed for use with patients with chronic fatigue syndrome. The Fatigue Severity Scale is a 7-point Likert scale that measures the impact of fatigue on daily functioning.[5] More than 20 self-report measures have been developed to measure fatigue in cancer. These scales are well described in tabular form in a recent review by well outlined in the review by Mitchell.[6]

PREVALENCE AND CAUSE OF CRF

The prevalence of CRF in the literature ranges between 25% and 99%.[7] In the setting of advanced cancer, almost 60% of patients experience fatigue.[8] CRF has been described with all cancer treatment modalities, including radiation, chemotherapy, and hematopoietic stem cell transplantation, hormonal and biologic treatments.[6] A complex interaction between various host and environmental stimuli are thought to contribute to CRF. Demographic variables associated with the severity and the occurrence of CRF include age, gender, and marital status. Numerous studies have shown an association with anemia, myeloid suppression, mood disorder, and concurrent symptoms, such as pain, electrolyte disturbances, medical comorbidities, deconditioning, medications (especially narcotics, which act on the central nervous system, may also contribute to fatigue).

Non-cancer comorbidities may contribute substantially to symptoms of fatigue in patients with cancer. One example would be anthracycline cardiomyopathy-related congestive heart failure. Heart failure is associated with significant fatigue and may be improved by optimizing that condition. Other comorbidities that need review and assessment include pulmonary, renal, hepatic, neurologic, and endocrine dysfunction, such as hypothyroidism, hypogonadism, adrenal insufficiency, and infection.

Sleep disturbance contribute to CRF. The relationship between sleep disturbance and CRF again bring into play a host of often reciprocal and interrelated systems, including altered circadian rhythms, proinflammatory cytokine activity, and abnormalities of the hypothalamic-pituitary axis. The contribution of sleep disorders to CRF symptoms and its mediators is the focus of much of the remainder of this article.

SLEEP DISTURBANCE

Sleep disturbances are common in patients with cancer. Up to 80% of patients with cancer will complain of sleep disturbance during diagnosis,

treatment, and as far as 10 years into survivorship. Daytime sleepiness and sleep disturbances have been reported to influence perceptions of fatigue.[9,10] A sleep disorder is defined as any disorder that affects, disrupts, or involves sleep. *The International Classification of Sleep Disorders, Second Edition*, provides a simple diagnostic framework that identifies 8 major categories of sleep disorders. These categories include insomnia; sleep-related breathing disorders, such as sleep apnea; hypersomnolence of central nervous system origin; circadian rhythm disorders; movement disorders; parasomnias; isolated symptoms/normal variants; and other disorders.[11] The terms hypersomnia and excessive daytime sleepiness (EDS) are often used synonymously. Sleep disorders may play an important role in the causation and pathophysiology of CRF. The role of sleep disorders and its effects on cancer and CRF are reviewed in the next few paragraphs.

SLEEP DISORDERS AND CANCER

Sleep duration and disturbed sleep are associated with increases in cancer risk. Early epidemiologic evidence for this was found in the increased incidence of breast cancer in long haul Finnish airline cabin attendants, who travel through multiple time zones and sleep discordantly with the internal circadian clock.[12] The investigators postulated that sleep discordant with the circadian clock or nonnocturnal sleep may contribute to the higher incidence of breast cancer in these women. This contribution is further strengthened by the recent epidemiologic studies demonstrating that the women working night shifts have a significantly elevated risk of breast,[13,20] endometrial,[14] and colorectal cancer.[15] Male night-shift workers were also at a significantly increased risk of developing prostate cancer, presumably because of their increased exposure to light at night.[16] Nocturnal darkness promotes nocturnal sleep in that darkness during the night is an absolute requirement for the production of melatonin. Melatonin has been shown in vitro and in vivo to have oncostatic properties, and the nocturnal surge of melatonin during dark nights represents a biologic timing signal that is internally driven by the activity of a central pacemaker in the suprachiasmatic nuclei. However, light exposure suppresses this melatonin expression by the pineal gland. There is up to a 5-fold higher risk of developing breast cancer in industrialized nations than in less developed countries, which may be, in part, because nocturnal light is common in the industrialized world.[17] Further evidence that rotating and nocturnal shift work may increase the risk of cancer derives from the Nurse's Health Study, which enrolled more than 70,000 respondents. This study found an increased relative risk (RR) of the incidence of breast cancer (RR = 1.4) in nurses who worked rotating shifts for more than 30 years. The low urine levels of melatonin metabolites found in these nurses is postulated to diminish melatonin's known potential oncostatic properties.[18,19] Alterations in circadian control of cell cycle genes may also play a role in oncogenesis. In part, circadian rhythms may have developed in unicellular organisms to limit DNA synthesis to periods when the cell would not be as exposed to the damaging influences of UV radiation from the sun.

There is increasing evidence to suggest that disturbed sleep has detrimental effects on the immune response. Cellular, hormonal, and inflammatory mediators are also affected by sleep disruption.[20] These data suggest a reciprocal relationship between sleep and immunity. Oncogenesis may be promoted in the setting of impaired immune system–mediated tumor surveillance and the proinflammatory milieu consequent to sleep disruption and abnormal circadian rhythms.[21]

Previous reports have demonstrated a high prevalence of sleep disturbance in patients with cancer.[10,22] Cytokine secretion has been shown to be disrupted and elevated in patients with breast cancer with sleep disturbance. Specifically, abnormalities of the secretion of the cytokines interleukin 6 (IL-6), tumor necrosis factor (TNF), and IL-1 have been demonstrated to correlate with sleep disturbances leading to insomnia, daytime sleepiness, and fatigue in both patients with cancer and patients without cancer.[23–25]

SLEEP AND CRF

Although CRF and cancer-related sleep disorders are distinct, a strong interrelationship exists between these symptoms, with a strong possibility that they may be reciprocally related. Most studies that have assessed both sleep and fatigue in patients with cancer provide evidence supporting a strong correlation between CRF and various sleep disorders, including poor sleep quality, disrupted initiation and maintenance of sleep, nighttime awakening, restless sleep, and EDS.[23,26] Many studies have come to the conclusion that "in cancer patients, sleep that is inadequate or unrefreshing may be important not only to the expression of fatigue, but to the patients' quality of life and their tolerance to treatment."[27] A recent study evaluated 20 adolescents undergoing chemotherapy and found a high correlation between sleep disturbance and CRF.[28] Sleep disturbance in CRF in many ways mimics the symptoms of fatigue with daytime lassitude similar to, although not identical, hypersomnia or EDS.

Some investigators have suggested that inflammatory changes related to cancer and cancer treatment may have a role in the clustering of symptoms of fatigue and sleep disturbance in these patients. Others have suggested the alteration of the circadian rhythms and desynchronized sleep-wake cycle may explain this relationship. The following paragraphs explain the inflammatory changes and the alteration in circadian rhythms of sleep and[29] wakefulness that may underlie these processes.

The literature regarding cytokines and sleep highlights. The role of the cytokines IL-1, IL-6 and TNF alpha is now understood to play a major role in regulating sleep disruption and fatigue. Both IL-1 and IL-6 can enhance slow wave non-rapid eye movement (NREM) sleep, and IL-1 may also affect the serotonergic pathway to increase NREM sleep. Human patients on IL-1 therapy often complain of fatigue and sleepiness. Recent studies suggest that IL-6 may be involved in the alteration of sleep, especially during illness. Under normal circumstances, IL-6 in plasma exhibits a diurnal rhythm with peak values during sleep and nadirs during wakefulness. Sleep deprivation of human patients increases IL-6, and subcutaneous injection of IL-6 increases slow-wave sleep and decreases REM sleep in humans. Patients with cancer, who are undergoing cancer therapy, experience significant alterations in their cytokine levels. These patients also experience the disabling symptoms of fatigue and sleepiness.[30,31] Furthermore, recent studies have also observed these associations in patients with metastatic breast cancer undergoing cancer therapy.[32] Bardwell[33] and Ancoli-Israel and colleagues[26] reviewed several reports that linked inflammatory cytokines to symptoms of fatigue and sleep disturbance. In addition, Savaard[26] demonstrated that these proinflammatory mediators, which were linked to fatigue and insomnia, improved with cognitive and behavioral therapy for insomnia (CBT-I).

Recently, it has been postulated that alterations in cytokine profiles may have direct effects on the neurobiology of sleep and the generation of circadian rhythms.[34,35] Furthermore, it is postulated that the central molecular clock through the suprachiasmatic nuclei directly influences the activation or inhibition of hypothalamic centers. This effect leads to altered cytokine and hormonal production, upsetting physiologic balance and resulting in symptoms such as sleep disturbance and fatigue.[36] Several recent studies have documented alteration in circadian rhythms in patients with breast cancer. Actigraphic evaluation of patients undergoing anthracycline- and paclitaxel (Taxol)-based che- motherapy for breast cancer reveals alterations in circadian rhythm variables in these patients.[37,38] Still other actigraphic studies have demonstrated that these changes in circadian rhythm can persist even 30 days after chemotherapy and that these abnormal rhythms correlate with an increased symptom burden of fatigue and sleepiness.[39] These data suggest that circadian rhythm distur- bance contributes to sleepiness and CRF in pa- tients with cancer.

MANAGEMENT OF CRF

Intervention for CRF must be multidimensional and individually tailored. General supportive care recommendations for treating CRF include opti- mizing nutritional status, preventing weight loss, and balancing rest with physical activity. There have been more than 170 empiric studies of phar- macologic and nonpharmacologic interventions to mitigate and manage CRF. Several recent meta-analyses and systematic reviews of the topic have been published.[30,40–42] Exercise, psychoedu- cational and self-management interventions, struc- tured rehabilitation, pharmacologic measures, treatment of anemia, and complimentary therapies have all been studied and are discussed in the next few paragraphs.

Meta-analyses of randomized trials provide findings to support the benefits of exercise in the management of CRF.[43,44] Exercise has been shown to improve aerobic capacity and decondi- tioning, prevent muscle loss, and may produce favorable effects on sleep. A variety of exercise modalities, including walking, cycling, swimming, resistive exercise, or a combination, have been studied. Further research is required to develop cancer-specific guidelines as to the intensity, na- ture, and safety of exercise in the treatment of CRF.

PSYCHOEDUCATIONAL AND SELF- MANAGEMENT INTERVENTIONS

There is considerable evidence the educational intervention and psychological improve CRF. En- ergy conservation and activity management (ECAM) is a self-management intervention that teaches patients to measure and balance energy use and provides support to incorporate these strategies into daily life. ECAM has been found to have a modest benefit in a large randomized controlled trial (RCT) involving mainly patients with breast cancer.[45] CBT-I, which incorporates sleep hygiene, behavioral modification, and an evaluation of attitudes and thoughts about sleep, has also been shown to improve sleep quality

and fatigue primarily in patients with breast can- cer.[26] A review by Zee and Ancoli-Israel[46] evalu- ated several studies of CBT-I in patients with cancer and noted improvements in sleep parame- ters as well as CRF.

Pharmacologic Interventions

Several pharmacologic agents, including antide- pressants, such as paroxetine, venlafaxine, and bupropion, as well as stimulant mediation, such as methylphenidate and modafinil, have been evaluated for their effectiveness in mitigating fatigue in patients with cancer. Trials with antide- pressants seem to indicate modest or no be- nefit for fatigue but improvement in depressive symptoms.[42]

The use of methylphenidate or dexmethylphe- nidate to reduce CRF has been evaluated in mul- tiple studies. Most (7 out of 9) RCTs support the benefit of these drugs. Side effects of these drugs include insomnia, agitation, anorexia, nausea, and vomiting.[6] Modafinil has been show in several trials to be effective in treating fatigue and im- proving daytime wakefulness and cognitive func- tion in patients with CRF.[47–49]

COMPLEMENTARY THERAPIES

Yoga, relaxation therapy, massage, and acupunc- ture have been used for the treatment of CRF. The studies evaluating these therapies are often small and uncontrolled. Further RCTs will be necessary to determine if these therapies may be used to treat CRF.[42]

RESEARCH ISSUES REGARDING SLEEP AND CRF

CRF continues to be a major concern of patients and providers of cancer care. The symptoms are debilitating and can persist many years after the cancer diagnosis and therapy. Further research is required to address the mechanisms of illness, including a better understanding of the complex interplay between the sleep system, circadian rhythms, inflammation, and the hypothalamic- pituitary axis. Genetic analysis and genomic studies need to be done to better understand which pa- tients may be prone to CRF and which therapies may exacerbate these symptoms. Additional inves- tigation is required into the question of which co- morbid conditions such as mood disturbance, anxiety disorders, physical deconditioning, cardio- vascular compromise, and endocrine dysfunction, contribute to CRF and sleep disturbance. Finally, more well-designed RCTs must be done to under- stand which modalities or perhaps multimodal therapies can be used to treat CRF. With the impetus coming from the large number of patients with these symptoms and with cancer diagnoses becoming more prevalent, the need for further research in CRF is pressing.

REFERENCES

1. Berger A, Abernathy A, Atkinsone A, et al. Cancer-related fatigue. J Natl Compr Canc Netw 2010;8: 904–31.

2. Cella D, Peterman A, Passik S, et al. Progress toward guidelines for the management of fatigue. Oncology 1998;12:369–77.

3. Yellen S, Cella D, Webster K. Measuring fatigue and other anemia-related symptoms with the Functional Assessment of Cancer Therapy (FACT) measurement system. J Pain Symptom Manage 1997;13(2): 63–74.

4. Chalder T, Berelowitz G, Pawlikowska T, et al. Development of a fatigue scale. J Psychosom Res 1993; 37:147–53.

5. Krupp L, LaRocca N, Muir-Nash J, et al. The fatigue severity scale. Application to patients with multiple sclerosis and systemic lupus erythematosus. Arch Neurol 1989;46:1121–3.

6. Mitchell S. Cancer-related fatigue: state of the science. PM R 2010;2:364–83.

7. Servaes P, Verhagen C, Bleijenberg G. Fatigue in cancer patients during and after treatment: prevalence, correlates and interventions. Eur J Cancer 2002;38:27–43.

8. Johnsen A, Peteren M, Pederen L. Symptoms and problems in a nationally representative sample of advanced cancer patients. Palliat Med 2009;23:491–501.

9. Berger AM, Mitchell SA. Modifying cancer-related fatigue by optimizing sleep quality. J Natl Compr Canc Netw 2008;6:3–13.

10. Savard J, Morin C. Insomnia in the context of cancer: a review of a neglected problem. J Clin Oncol 2001;19:895–908.

11. American Academy of Sleep Medicine. International classification of sleep disorders, 2nd ed.: diagnostic and coding manual. Westchester (IL): American Academy of Sleep Medicne; 2005.

12. Kojo K, Pukkala E, Auvinen A. Breast cancer risk among Finnish cabin attendants: a nested case-control study. Occup Environ Med 2005;62.488–93.

13. Davis S, Mirick DK, Stevens RG. Night shift work, light at night, and risk of breast cancer. J Natl Cancer Inst 2001;93:1557–62.

14. Viswanathan AN, Hankinson SE, Schernhammer ES. Night –shift work and the risk of endometrial cancer. Cancer Res 2007;67:10618–22.

15. Schernhammer ES, Laden F, Speizer FE, et al. Night-shift work and the risk of colorectal cancer in the nurses' health study. J Natl Cancer Inst 2003;95:825–8.

16. Kubo T, Ozasa K, Mikami K, et al. Prospective cohort study of the risk of prostate cancer among rotating –shift workers: finding form the Japan collaborative cohort. Am J Epidemiol 2006;164: 549–55.

17. Stevens RG. Electrical power use and breast cancer: a hypothesis. Am J Epidemiol 1987;125:556–61.

18. Schernhammer ES, Schulmeister K. Melatonin and cancer risk: does light and night compromise physiologic cancer protection by lowering serum melatonin levels? Br J Cancer 2004;90:941–3.

19. Schernhammer ES, Laden F, Speizer FE, et al. Rotating night shifts and risk of breast cancer in woman participating in the nurses' health study. J Natl Cancer Inst 2001;93:1563–8.

20. Born J, Lange T, Hansen K, et al. Effects of sleep and circadian rhythms on human circulating immune cells. J Immunol 1997;158:4454–64.

21. Bryant PA, Trinder J, Curtis N. Sick and tired: does sleep have a vital role in the immune system? Nat Rev Immunol 2004;4:457–67.

22. Davidson JR, Waisberg JL, Brundage MD, et al. Nonpharmacologic group treatment of insomnia: a preliminary study with cancer survivors. Psychoon-cology 2001;10:389–97.

23. Vgontzas A, Chrousos G. Sleep, the hypothalamic-pituitary-adrenal axis, and cytokines: multiple interaction and disturbances in sleep disorders. Endocrinol Metab Clin North Am 2002;31:15–36.

24. Fiorentino L, Ancoli-Israel S. Insomnia and its treatment in women with breast cancer. Sleep Med Rev 2006;10:419–29.

25. Savard S, Ivers M. Randomized study on the efficacy of cognitive and behavioral therapy for insomnia secondary to breast cancer, part I: sleep and psychological effects. J Clin Oncol 2005; 23(25):6083–96.

26. Ancoli-Israel S, Moore PJ, Jones V. The relationship between fatigue and sleep in cancer patients: a review. Eur J Cancer Care (Engl) 2001; 10:245–55.

27. Roscoe JA, Kaufman ME, Matteson-Rusby SE, et al. Cancer-related fatigue and sleep disorders. Oncologist 2007;12(Suppl 1):35–42.

28. Erickson J, Beck S, Christian B. Fatigue, sleep-wake disturbances, and quality of life in adolescents receiving chemotherapy. J Pediatr Hematol Oncol 2011;33.e17–25.

29. Mitchell S, Beck S, Hood L. Putting evidence into practice (PEP): evidence-based interventions for fatigue during and following cancer and its treatment. Clin J Oncol Nurs 2007;11(1):99–113.

30. Wood LJ. Cancer Chemotherapy-related symptoms: evidence to suggest a role for pro-inflammatory cytokines. Oncol Nurs Forum 2006;33:535–42.

31. Vena C, Parker K, Cunningham M. Sleep-wake disturbances in people with cancer part I: an

overview of sleep, sleep regulation, and effects of disease and treatment. Oncol Nurs Forum 2004; 31:735–46.

32. Payne J. Biomarkers, fatigue, sleep and depressive symptoms in women with breast cancer: a pilot study. Oncol Nurs Forum 2006;33:775–83.

33. Bardwell WA, Ancoli-Israel S. Breast Cancer and Fatigue. Sleep Med Clin 2008;3(1):61–71.

34. Kapsimalis F, Basta M, Varouchakis G, et al. Cytokines and pathological sleep. Sleep 2008;9: 603–14.

35. Imeri L, Opp MR. How (and why) the immune system makes us sleep. Nat Rev Neurosci 2009;10:199–210.

36. Hastings MH, Herzog ED. Clock genes, oscillators, and cellular networks in the suprachiasmatic nuclei. J Biol Rhythms 2004;19(5):400–1.

37. Savard L, Rissling N, He D, et al. Breast cancer patients have progressively impaired sleep-wake activity rhythms during chemotherapy. Sleep 2009;32(9): 1155–60.

38. Roscoe J, Kaufman ME, Mattsen SE, et al. Cancer related fatigue and sleep disorders. Oncologist 2008;12(Suppl):35–42.

39. Berger AM, Wielgus K, Hertzog M, et al. Patterns of circadian activity rhythms and their relationships with fatigue and anxiety/depression in women treated with breast cancer adjuvant chemotherapy. Support Care Cancer 2010;18(1):105–14.

40. Kangas M, Bovbjerg D, Mongomery G. Cancer-related fatigue: a systematic and meta-analytic review of the non-pharmacological therapies for cancer patients. Psychol Bull 2008;134:700–41.

41. Minton O, Richardson A, Sharpe M. A systematic review and meta-analysis of the pharmacological treatment of cancer-related fatigue.

42. Jacobson P, Donovan K, Vadaparampil ST. Systematic review and meta-analysis of psychological and activity-based interventions for cancer-related fatigue. Health Psychol 2007;26:660–7.

43. Cramp F, Daniel J. Exercise for the management of cancer-related fatigue in adults. Cochrane Database Syst Rev 2008;(2):CD006145.

44. Conn V, Hafdahl A, Porock D. A meta-analysis of exercise interventions among people with cancer. Support Care Cancer 2006;14:699–712.

45. Barsevick A, Dudley W, Beck S. A randomized clinical trial of energy conservation for patients with cancer-related fatigue. Cancer 2004;100:1302–10.

46. Zee P, Ancoli-Israel S. Does effective management of sleep disorders reduce cancer-related fatigue? Drugs 2009;69(Suppl 2):29–41.

47. Blackhall L, Petroni G, Shu J. A pilot study evaluating the safety and efficacy of modafinil for cancer-related fatigue. J Palliat Med 2009;12:433–9.

48. Cooper M, Bird H, Steinberg M. Efficacy and safety of modafinil in the treatment of cancer –related fatigue. Ann Pharmacother 2009;43:721–5.

49. Spathis A, Dhillan R, Booden D. Modafinil for the treatment of fatigue in lung cancer: a pilot study. Palliat Med 2009;23:325–31.

Sleep Disorders and Fatigue

Sheila C. Tsai, MD*, Teofilo Lee-Chiong Jr, MD

KEYWORDS

- Fatigue • Narcolepsy • Sleepiness • Sleep disorders • Insomnia

KEY POINTS

- Fatigue is a prominent symptom in numerous medical disorders.
- Many individuals with cardiovascular, endocrine, psychiatric, and neurologic disorders experience significant, sometimes debilitating, fatigue.
- Although several sleep disorders are characterized by pathologic sleepiness, fatigue can be a major symptom in some sleep disorders.
- Identifying and managing underlying sleep disorders may improve sleep and attenuate fatigue.

Fatigue is defined by a lack of energy or a sensation of tiredness that may improve with rest. It is essential to distinguish fatigue from sleepiness. Fatigue can be described as lack of energy or weariness. Sleepiness, on the other hand, is commonly associated with inattention, constant yawning, frequent lapses into sleep, or struggling to stay awake. One important difference between fatigue and sleepiness is that the former may improve with rest alone and without sleep, whereas the latter worsens with resting or remaining sedentary.[1]

Fatigue is a prominent symptom in many disease conditions, and about 20% of visits to family practice physicians are related to complaints of fatigue.[2] Fatigue is frequently a predominant or associated symptom in mood disorders, particularly anxiety or depression. Conversely, depressive and anxiety symptoms are risk factors for new-onset or persistent fatigue among adolescents.[3–5]

The etiology of fatigue is not clear. Proposed mechanisms include cortisol imbalance[6] and release of inflammatory mediators.[7] Fatigue is associated with many disease states, such as cardiovascular disease, endocrine abnormalities, multiple sclerosis, and sickness behavior, that are associated with an increased inflammatory state.[8–10] Sickness behavior, characterized by a constellation of symptoms (decreased appetite, anhedonia, decreased pain tolerance, psychomotor slowing, and fatigue), occurs after exposure to pathogens or cytokine administration (ie, the common manifestations in individuals who are ill from microbial infections).[8] It is this enhanced inflammatory state and altered immunomodulation that may be the pathogenetic link between sleep disorders and fatigue.

Rating scales have attempted to objectively quantify and categorize subjective complaints of fatigue. One commonly used scale is the Fatigue Severity Scale (FSS).[11] The FSS consists of a series of 7 questions regarding fatigue that are rated from 1 to 9. A score of 36 or greater is considered positive for the presence of fatigue.

SLEEP DISORDERS AND FATIGUE

As stated earlier, it is important to properly characterize fatigue and sleepiness when obtaining a medical history from patients suspected of having a sleep disorder. Sleepiness is a prominent clinical feature of many sleep disorders including insufficient sleep syndrome, narcolepsy, obstructive sleep apnea (OSA), and circadian rhythm sleep disorders, such as shift work disorder (SWD). In these sleep disorders, patients commonly complain of

National Jewish Health, University of Colorado Denver School of Medicine, 1400 Jackson Street, Denver, CO 80206, USA
* Corresponding author. National Jewish Health, 1400 Jackson Street, G012, Denver, CO 80206, USA.
E-mail address: tsais@njhealth.org

Sleep Med Clin 8 (2013) 235–239
http://dx.doi.org/10.1016/j.jsmc.2013.02.003

difficulty staying awake and may fall asleep unintentionally. Importantly, sleepiness improves following appropriate therapy (eg, sleep extension for insufficient sleep syndrome, psychostimulants for narcolepsy and idiopathic hypersomnia, and positive airway pressure therapy for OSA).

Sleep disorders may also give rise to fatigue. In addition to the sleep disorders already mentioned, chronic sleep deprivation can result in fatigue and lack of motivation. Also, fatigue, either in lieu of, or in addition to sleepiness, is a prominent feature of insomnia and restless legs syndrome (RLS).

INSOMNIA

Insomnia refers to difficulty falling asleep, staying asleep, and/or nonrestorative sleep. It is associated with daytime impairments resulting from poor sleep.[12] Patients with insomnia often describe feeling physically or mentally tired or fatigued but often do not complain of sleepiness.[13] Imaging studies in patients with insomnia have demonstrated relative increased activity in certain brain regions during sleep, as well as areas of decreased activity during wake.[14] This suggests that fatigue may arise from inappropriate arousability during the sleep period and reduced brain metabolic activity during waking. In addition, it has been theorized that insomnia is associated with chronic psychophysiologic hyperarousal.[15,16] Finally, comorbid depression, anxiety, or psychological distress is common in insomnia and may adversely impact daytime functioning.[17]

Excessive anxiety regarding sleep may be a better predictor of daytime fatigue than objective sleep parameters. Perceptions about inadequate sleep duration and poor sleep quality can influence the severity of fatigue complaints. Decreases in slow wave sleep, rapid eye movement (REM) sleep, and total sleep time often accompany sleep fragmentation.[18] Sleep fragmentation may result in more complaints of exhaustion and sleepiness, that, in turn, can lead to less physical activity. Thus, sleep quality, rather than sleep quantity, may be a more important factor in the development of fatigue in patients with insomnia. However, both subjective sleep quality and objective measures of sleep are important; in one study, among persons with similar levels of fatigue, those with more severe objective sleep disruption reported lower quality-of-life scores.[19]

OBSTRUCTIVE SLEEP APNEA

OSA is a form of sleep-disordered breathing characterized by repetitive cessation (apnea) or reduction (hypopnea) of respiration due to complete (apnea) or partial (hypopnea) upper airway obstruction during sleep. OSA, if left untreated, can produce cardiovascular and neurocognitive consequences, in addition to excessive sleepiness and fatigue.[20] Daytime sleepiness and mental fatigue are associated with a higher risk of accidents due to lapses in alertness or vigilance.[21,22]

Compared with hypersomnia, the association between OSA and fatigue is not as well defined. It is unclear what factors or mechanisms contribute to development of fatigue in persons with OSA. Although fatigue can certainly result from sleep fragmentation and chronic sleep deprivation, studies have demonstrated that fatigue in OSA is more closely correlated with severity of depressive symptoms rather than severity of OSA.[23] Depressive symptoms contribute up to 50% of the variance in fatigue in OSA patients, a value 10 times higher than that contributed by OSA severity.[24,25] About half of patients with OSA have at least mild depression[26,27] and almost 20% may be classified as having major depressive disorder.[28] Thus, OSA can give rise to fatigue directly via sleep disruption or indirectly by its interactions with depressive symptoms. Lastly, perceived sleep quality appears to be just as important as objective measures of sleep in predicting fatigue.[17]

Treatment with positive airway pressure (PAP) remains the therapy of choice for most patients with OSA. However, despite treatment with PAP devices, some patients with OSA may suffer from persistent sleepiness and fatigue. In these patients, it is important to exclude suboptimal therapy, noncompliance, significant increases in weight, or development of new sleep or medical disorders that can give rise to fatigue.[29]

RESTLESS LEGS SYNDROME

Persons with RLS report an uncomfortable sensation or urge to move the legs and sometimes the arms. It is worse at rest and in the evening and is usually relieved by movement. RLS affects about 5% to 15% of the population.[30] It causes sleep disruption and has been associated with fatigue. The latter may arise from increased inflammation caused by significant sleep disruption and comorbid depression. Complaints of lack of energy and tendency for depression have been noted in about 60% and 54% of affected individuals, respectively.[31] This high associated rate for depression may account for an increase in fatigue complaints. Older adults with RLS symptoms have significantly higher depression scores compared with those without RLS.[32] Furthermore, insomnia is common among patients with RLS and may also contribute to the development of fatigue. Severe RLS is associated with both poorer sleep quality, as measured using the Pittsburgh Sleep Quality Index (PSQI), and reduced sleep quantity.[33] Patients with RLS commonly have worse quality-of-life scores, with ratings similar to those with other chronic medical conditions.

By worsening sleep quality, RLS may exacerbate fatigue in certain chronic disorders, such as multiple sclerosis (MS) and diabetes mellitus (DM). In persons with type 2 DM, the presence of RLS is associated with worse sleep quality (PSQI scores), longer sleep onset latency, more daytime complaints, more depression, and greater fatigue (higher FSS scores).[34] Similarly, RLS negatively affects sleep quality in persons with MS and can increase the likelihood and severity of fatigue. In 1 study, the prevalence of RLS among patients with MS was 27%. Individuals with both MS and RLS note poorer sleep quality and higher levels of fatigue than in MS without RLS.[35]

Individuals with fibromyalgia (FM) generally have more complaints of sleepiness, fatigue, and insomnia than the general population.[1] They also have a higher prevalence of RLS; in 1 study, RLS was 10 times more prevalent among patients with FM than in controls.[36] Treatment of RLS, if present, may improve sleep quality and quality of life in patients with FM.

SHIFT WORK

Up to 25% of the US workforce has a nontraditional work schedule, working evening, rotating, or night shifts.[37] This high number of shift workers is related to the increased connectedness of the world, the global nature of the economy, and 24-hour communication. Shift work disorder (SWD) is characterized by insomnia, excessive sleepiness, or both. In SWD, the worker's endogenous circadian rhythm is desynchronized from the required work schedules, since they are expected to work during typical sleep times, and sleep during typical wake times.

While sleepiness is a key feature of SWD, fatigue is also associated with shift work. Shift workers suffer from more fatigue-related accidents. About 30% to 40% of truck accidents are considered fatigue-related.[1] When evaluating shift workers and their complaints of fatigue, the frequency of shift work affected symptoms of subjective fatigue.[37] The mean FSS score increased as the frequency of shift work increased. When comparing shift workers to nonshift workers, those with 3 or more shifts per week had higher FSS scores. The most fatigued patients also objectively had the worst sleep quality with lower nocturnal oxygen

saturations and worse sleep efficiencies. Interestingly, sleepiness and fatigue did not correlate with each other. In this study, the severity of fatigue experienced by the shift workers was similar to the severity of fatigue in those with chronic diseases such as MS and lupus.

Medical personnel, including nurses, frequently engage in shift work. Among nurses, both working more shifts and having more frequent shifts increase severity of fatigue.[38] In this group, poor sleep quality is the factor most closely associated with complaints of fatigue.[39,40] Anxiety and mood disorders also play a role in fatigue among these shift workers.

Various mechanisms for the fatigue noted in shift workers have been proposed. In contrast to normal individuals, in whom cortisol levels are highest upon awakening in the morning and decrease over the course of the day, morning cortisol levels were lower in night shift nurses than in their day shift counterparts.[38] It has been theorized that high cortisol concentrations and low melatonin levels during the day contribute to difficulty sleeping and poor sleep quality following night shifts. Fatigue may also be related to chronic sleep loss, circadian desynchrony, and comorbid sleep disorders.[41] It is estimated that 70% of fatigued shift workers have an underlying coexisting sleep disorder, such as OSA or RLS.[36]

NARCOLEPSY

Narcolepsy is a neurologic disorder characterized by chronic excessive daytime sleepiness. Other associated features include cataplexy, sleep paralysis, sleep hallucinations, and sleep disturbance. Patients with narcolepsy also often have significant fatigue.[42] Using the Checklist Individual Strength (CIS) test as a measure of fatigue, investigators have reported a prevalence of severe fatigue of 62.5% in patients with narcolepsy. Fatigue in this population was associated with greater functional impairment, more depressive symptoms, and worse quality of life. Interestingly, fatigued and nonfatigued subjects did not differ in subjective sleepiness as determined using the Epworth sleepiness scale. Use of stimulant medications was greater among fatigued subjects compared with those without fatigue.[43]

Many patients with narcolepsy–cataplexy possess the human leukocyte antigen (HLA) DQB1*0602 allele. Positivity for this allele may explain, in part, differences in fatigue, sleepiness, and sleep requirements among healthy individuals.[44] Treatment with modafinil for excessive sleepiness has also been shown to reduce fatigue and improve vigor in patients with narcolepsy.[45]

NEUROLOGIC DISORDERS

Sleep quality and duration play important roles in the development and progression of fatigue in several chronic neurologic conditions. Among patients with traumatic brain injuries (TBIs), poor sleep and anxiety were among the top 3 most important independent factors associated with fatigue.[46]

Fatigue is a major feature of MS and negatively impacts quality of life. In these patients, fatigue is related, in large part, to inflammatory mediators. In addition, medications used to treat MS and depression can contribute to fatigue. Patients with MS often complain of sleep disturbance and poor sleep quality, and have higher rates of chronic insomnia. These sleep problems, in turn, may worsen underlying fatigue.[47] Due to disruption of dopaminergic pathways, patients with MS may experience RLS. The presence of RLS can, as mentioned previously, worsen fatigue. Finally, patients with MS may have higher risks for central sleep apnea and OSA, both of which can lead to fatigue.

Poor sleep quality, including reduced total sleep times, decreased sleep efficiency, and increased prevalence of sleep apnea can contribute to fatigue in patients with amyotrophic lateral sclerosis (ALS).[48] Conversely, ALS patients with fatigue can experience more difficulty with sleep, have more problems with staying asleep, and report more nocturnal complaints than ALS patients without fatigue.

SUMMARY

Fatigue is a prominent symptom in numerous disorders. Many individuals with cardiovascular, endocrine, psychiatric (anxiety and depression), and neurologic (MS) disorders complain of significant, sometimes debilitating, fatigue. Although several sleep disorders are characterized by pathologic sleepiness, fatigue can also be a major factor in some sleep disorders. A good sleep history, including sleep quality, sleep quantity, work schedule, and perceptions regarding sleep is needed when patients present with complaints of fatigue. Identifying and managing underlying sleep disorders may help attenuate the fatigue experienced by these patients. Improving sleep may also reduce the severity of fatigue in persons suffering from other chronic underlying disorders.

REFERENCES

1. Akerstedt T, Wright KP Jr. Sleep loss and fatigue in shift work and shift work disorder. Sleep Med Clin 2009;4(2):257–71.
2. Rosenthal TC, Majeroni BA, Pretorius R, et al. Fatigue: an overview. Am Fam Physician 2008;78(10):1173–9.
3. Rimes KA, Goodman R, Hotopf M, et al. Incidence, prognosis, and risk factors for fatigue and chronic fatigue syndrome in adolescents: a prospective community study. Pediatrics 2007;119(3):e603–9.
4. Viner RM, Clark C, Taylor SJ, et al. Longitudinal risk factors for persistent fatigue in adolescents. Arch Pediatr Adolesc Med 2008;162(5):469–75.
5. ter Wolbeek M, van Doornen LJ, Kavelaars A, et al. Predictors of persistent and new-onset fatigue in adolescent girls. Pediatrics 2008;121(3):449–57.
6. Kudielka BM, Buchtal J, Uhde A, et al. Circadian cortisol profiles and psychological self-reports in shift workers with and without recent change in the shift rotation system. Biol Psychol 2007;74(1):92–103.
7. Dehghan A, Dupuis J, Barbalic M, et al. Meta-analysis of genome-wide association studies in >80 000 subjects identifies multiple loci for C-reactive protein levels. Circulation 2011;123(7):731–8.
8. Dantzer R. Cytokine-induced sickness behavior: where do we stand? Brain Behav Immun 2001;15(1):7–24.
9. Chawla A, Nguyen KD, Goh YP. Macrophage-mediated inflammation in metabolic disease. Nat Rev Immunol 2011;11(11):738–49.
10. Lurie A. Inflammation, oxidative stress, and procoagulant and thrombotic activity in adults with obstructive sleep apnea. Adv Cardiol 2011;46:43–66.
11. Krupp LB, LaRocca NG, Muir-Nash J, et al. The fatigue severity scale. Application to patients with multiple sclerosis and systemic lupus erythematosus. Arch Neurol 1989;46(10):1121–3.
12. American Academy of Sleep Medicine. Insomnia. The international classification of sleep disorders, 2nd edition: diagnostic and coding manual. Westchester (IL): American Academy of Sleep Medicine; 2005. p. 1–2.
13. Riedel BW, Lichstein KL. Insomnia and daytime functioning. Sleep Med Rev 2000;4(3):277–98.
14. Nofzinger EA, Buysse DJ, Germain A, et al. Functional neuroimaging evidence for hyperarousal in insomnia. Am J Psychiatry 2004;161(11):2126–8.
15. Riemann D, Spiegelhalder K, Feige B, et al. The hyperarousal model of insomnia: a review of the concept and its evidence. Sleep Med Rev 2010;14(1):19–31.
16. Bonnet MH, Arand DL. Hyperarousal and insomnia: state of the science. Sleep Med Rev 2010;14(1):9–15.
17. Fortier-Brochu E, Beaulieu-Bonneau S, Ivers H, et al. Relations between sleep, fatigue, and health-related quality of life in individuals with insomnia. J Psychosom Res 2010;69(5):475–83.
18. Hursel R. Effects of sleep fragmentation in healthy men on energy expenditure, substrate oxidation, physical activity, and exhaustion measured over

48 h in a respiratory chamber. Am J Clin Nutr 2011; 94(3):804–8.

19. Pilcher JJ, Ginter DR, Sadowsky B. Sleep quality versus sleep quantity: relationships between sleep and measures of health, well-being and sleepiness in college students. J Psychosom Res 1997;42(6): 583–96.

20. Monahan K, Redline S. Role of obstructive sleep apnea in cardiovascular disease. Curr Opin Cardiol 2011;26(6):541–7.

21. Mitler MM, Carskadon MA, Czeisler CA, et al. Catastrophes, sleep and public policy: consensus report. Sleep 1988;11(1):100–9.

22. George CF. Sleep. 5: driving and automobile crashes in patients with obstructive sleep apnoea/hypopnoea syndrome. Thorax 2004;59(9):804–7.

23. Stepnowsky CJ, Palau JJ, Zamora T, et al. Fatigue in sleep apnea: the role of depressive symptoms and self-reported sleep quality. Sleep Med 2011;12(9): 832–7.

24. Bardwell WA, Moore P, Ancoli-Israel S, et al. Fatigue in obstructive sleep apnea: driven by depressive symptoms instead of apnea severity? Psychiatry 2003;160(2):350–5.

25. Jackson ML, Stough C, Howard ME, et al. The contribution of fatigue and sleepiness to depression in patients attending the sleep laboratory for evaluation of obstructive sleep apnea. Sleep Breath 2010; 15(3):439–45.

26. Kales A, Caldwell AB, Cadieux RJ, et al. Severe obstructive sleep apnea–II: associated psychopathology and psychosocial consequences. J Chronic Dis 1985;38(5):427–34.

27. McCall WV, Harding D, O'Donovan C. Correlates of depressive symptoms in patients with obstructive sleep apnea. J Clin Sleep Med 2006;2(4):424–6.

28. Ohayon MM. The effects of breathing-related sleep disorders on mood disturbances in the general population. J Clin Psychiatry 2003;64(10): 1195–200.

29. Guilleminault C, Philip P. Tiredness and somnolence despite initial treatment of obstructive sleep apnea syndrome (what to do when an OSAS patient stays hypersomnolent despite treatment). Sleep 1996; 19(Suppl 9):S117–22.

30. Yeh P, Walters AS, Tsuang JW. Restless legs syndrome: a comprehensive overview on its epidemiology, risk factors, and treatment. Sleep Breath 2012;16:987–1007.

31. Hening W, Walters AS, Allen RP, et al. Impact, diagnosis and treatment of restless legs syndrome (RLS) in a primary care population: the REST (RLS epidemiology, symptoms, and treatment) primary care study. Sleep Med 2004;5:237–46.

32. Rothdach AJ, Trenkwalder C, Haberstock J, et al. Prevalence and risk factors of RLS in an elderly population: the MEMO study. Neurology 2000;54: 1064–8.

33. Cuellar NG, Strumpf NE, Ratcliffe SJ. Symptoms of restless legs syndrome in older adults: outcomes on sleep quality, sleepiness, fatigue, depression, and quality of life. J Am Geriatr Soc 2007;55(9): 1387–92.

34. Cuellar NG, Ratcliffe SJ. A comparison of glycemic control, sleep, fatigue, and depression in type 2 diabetes with and without restless legs syndrome. J Clin Sleep Med 2008;4(1):50–6.

35. Moreira NC, Damasceno RS, Medeiros CA, et al. Restless leg syndrome, sleep quality and fatigue in multiple sclerosis patients. Braz J Med Biol Res 2008;41(10):932–7.

36. Viola-Saltzman M, Watson NF, Bogart A, et al. High prevalence of restless legs syndrome among patients with fibromyalgia: a controlled cross-sectional study. J Clin Sleep Med 2010;6(5):423–7.

37. Shen J, Botly LC, Chung SA, et al. Fatigue and shift work. J Sleep Res 2006;15(1):1–5.

38. Niu SF, Chung MH, Chen CH, et al. The effect of shift rotation on employee cortisol profile, sleep quality, fatigue, and attention level: a systematic review. J Nurs Res 2011;19(1):68–81.

39. Samaha E, Lal S, Samaha N, et al. Psychological, lifestyle and coping contributors to chronic fatigue in shift-worker nurses. J Adv Nurs 2007;59(3):221–32.

40. Ruggiero JS. Correlates of fatigue in critical care nurses. Res Nurs Health 2003;26(6):434–44.

41. Muecke S. Effects of rotating night shifts: literature review. J Adv Nurs 2005;50(4):433–9.

42. Schneider C, Fulda S, Schulz H. Daytime variation in performance and tiredness/sleepiness ratings in patients with insomnia, narcolepsy, sleep apnea and normal controls. J Sleep Res 2004;13(4):373–83.

43. Droogleever Fortuyn HA, Fronczek R, Smitshoek M, et al. Severe fatigue in narcolepsy with cataplexy. J Sleep Res 2012;21(2):163–9.

44. Goel N, Banks S, Mignot E, et al. DQB1*0602 predicts interindividual differences in physiologic sleep, sleepiness, and fatigue. Neurology 2010;75(17): 1509–19.

45. Becker PM, Schwartz JR, Feldman NT, et al. Effect of modafinil on fatigue, mood, and health-related quality of life in patients with narcolepsy. Psychopharmacology (Berl) 2004;171(2):133–9.

46. Schnleders J, Willemsen D, de Boer H. Factors contributing to chronic fatigue after traumatic brain injury. J Head Trauma Rehabil 2012;27:404–12.

47. Braley TJ, Chervin RD. Fatigue in multiple sclerosis: mechanisms, evaluation, and treatment. Sleep 2010; 33(8):1061–7.

48. Lo Coco D, La Bella V. Fatigue, sleep, and nocturnal complaints in patients with amyotrophic lateral sclerosis. Eur J Neurol 2012;19(5):760–3.

Fatigue in Other Medical Disorders

Hashir Majid, MD[a],*, Munira Shabbir-Moosajee, MD[a],
Sarah Nadeem, MD[b]

KEYWORDS

- Fatigue • Chronic kidney disease • Endocrine disorders • Anemia • Parathyroid • Thyroid
- Hematological disorders • Cancer

KEY POINTS

- Fatigue associated with medical disorders can have a significant impact on functional status, quality of life, and clinical outcomes.
- A variety of medical diseases can be associated with fatigue, including renal, hematological, and endocrine pathologies.
- The pathophysiology of fatigue and sleepiness in the setting of some common medical problems is discussed in this review.
- Treatment focuses on correction of the underlying medical disorder.

We review fatigue and sleepiness caused by renal, hematological, and endocrine diseases in this article.

RENAL DISORDERS

Both acute and chronic kidney disease are associated with symptoms of fatigue, lethargy, and malaise.[1,2] There is no specific treatment for fatigue in renal diseases. Management focuses on treating the underlying etiology of the kidney disease and preventing progression of renal dysfunction, if possible. Supportive measures, including medical therapy and dialysis, may need to be initiated. Because most available data pertain to symptoms in chronic renal failure, most of this section focuses on fatigue in chronic kidney disease (CKD).

FATIGUE IN CHRONIC KIDNEY DISEASE

Fatigue is the initial and one of the cardinal manifestations of CKD.[1,3] This is irrespective of the etiology of CKD. Unlike healthy individuals, in whom fatigue can be a protective mechanism aimed at

obtaining rest and replenishment to overcome physical and mental stress, fatigue in medical disorders can be severely debilitating.[4] In CKD, it has significant impact on quality of life and is associated with substantial morbidity and mortality.[5,6]

CKD is divided into 5 stages based on the glomerular filtration rate (GFR).[7] The initial stages (stages 1 and 2) are mostly asymptomatic. Clinical manifestations, including fatigue, generally first become apparent with a drop in GFR below 60 mL/min/1.73 m^2 (stage 3 CKD). Symptoms are generally progressive unless appropriate management of CKD is initiated. Even with optimal therapy, many patients continue to experience malaise/fatigue.

The pathogenesis of fatigue in CKD is multifactorial. Anemia, disordered calcium and phosphate metabolism, wasting, and depression are all implicated (see **Table 1**).[8]

Anemia in Chronic Kidney Disease

Anemia is common in patients with CKD.[9] More than half of patients with advanced-stage CKD have low hemoglobin levels.[10]

The authors have no conflicts of interest to disclose.
[a] Department of Medicine, Aga Khan University, PO Box 3500, 1st Floor, FOB Building, Karachi 74800, Pakistan;
[b] Dreyer Medical Clinic, 1870 W Galena Boulevard, Aurora, IL 60506, USA
* Corresponding author.
E-mail address: hashir.majid@aku.edu

Sleep Med Clin 8 (2013) 241–253
http://dx.doi.org/10.1016/j.jsmc.2013.02.007

Table 1
Factors contributing to fatigue in CKD

	Mechanisms	Management Strategy
Anemia	Decreased erythropoietin levels, blood loss, iron deficiency, and disturbed iron homeostasis, shortened RBC life span	Erythropoiesis stimulating agents Iron supplementation
Mineral and bone disorder	Phosphate retention due to decreased GFR, secondary hypothyroidism, Vitamin D deficiency	Vitamin D supplementation Phosphate dietary restriction Phosphate binders
Protein energy wasting	Decreased oral intake, increased metabolic rate, catabolic state, inability to use free amino acids, insulin resistance, deranged appetite hormones	Nutritional supplements Correction of metabolic acidosis
Depression	Proinflammatory state, poor quality of life, disruption of social life, comorbid conditions	Nonpharmacologic treatment Cautious use of antidepressants
Uremia/Uremic milieu[a]	Increased nitrogenous waste products, systemic inflammation and altered cytokine state, increased oxidant stress	Treatment of underlying cause of renal disease Dialysis

Abbreviations: GFR, glomerular filtration rate; RBC, red blood cell.
[a] Uremia/uremic milieu is thought to be the major mechanism of fatigue in acute kidney failure.

The major mechanism for CKD-associated anemia is decreased erythropoietin (EPO) production from the renal interstitial fibroblasts adjacent to the peritubular capillaries.[11–13] Decreased glomerular filtration rate with advancing renal disease, leading to depletion and injury of EPO-producing cells, is the postulated cause for EPO deficiency. EPO enhances red cell production by its stimulatory effect on erythroid progenitor cells and by inhibiting apoptosis of these cells. Deficiency of EPO leads to ineffective erythropoiesis. EPO also has been shown to have neuroprotective properties in animal models.[14–17] Whether this has any contribution to the fatigue experienced by patients with CKD, and, related to this, improvement in fatigue symptoms with treatment of anemia with recombinant EPO is unknown.

Other causes of anemia include blood loss, iron deficiency, "uremic milieu," and diminished half-life of red blood cells in patients with CKD.[13] Blood loss is thought to be attributable to the well-known platelet dysfunction observed in patients with CKD and occurs predominantly in patients on hemodialysis. Iron loss is up to 20-fold higher in these patients when compared with healthy individuals and contributes to a state of iron deficiency. Decreased transferrin levels and sequestration of iron in the reticulo-endothelial system also occur in CKD and, along with accelerated iron losses, lead to abnormal iron homeostasis resulting in iron-deficiency anemia. The "uremic milieu," which is postulated to suppress erythroid progenitor cells, along with shortened RBC half-life in patients on hemodialysis, contributes to the development

of anemia. The net effect is that anemia becomes more and more prevalent with advancing stages of CKD: from about 5% and 44% in stages 3 and 4 respectively, to almost universal in stage 5 CKD.[18]

Calcium, Phosphate Metabolism

Abnormal calcium and phosphate levels have been associated with fatigue in CKD.[8] They have also been associated with elevated cardiovascular events and mortality.[19–22] Glomerular filtration rate, tubular reabsorption, vitamin D, parathyroid hormone (PTH), and fibroblast growth factor 23 (FGF 23) are the main determinants of calcium and phosphate metabolism in CKD.[23]

A declining filtered load of phosphate makes patients with CKD prone to development of hyperphosphatemia.[24] Hypersecretion of fibroblast growth factor (FGF)-23 and PTH in initial stages of CKD is successful in maintaining calcium and phosphate homeostasis. This is achieved by enhancement of urinary phosphate excretion (under the effect of both FGF-23 and PTH), along with release of calcium from the bones under the influence of PTH to correct the hypocalcemia of CKD (see later in this article).

Once the GFR falls below 40 mL/min, however, the compensatory mechanisms are overwhelmed and phosphate retention becomes a significant problem unless addressed with dietary restriction and medications.[25] In addition, the hypersecretion of FGF-23 and PTH can itself lead to worsening of phosphate concentrations: calcium release from bones under PTH is accompanied by phosphate liberation, whereas high FGF-23 levels can also affect bone mineralization.

Vitamin D and calcium metabolism are also affected in CKD. Both vitamin D deficiency and hypocalcemia may themselves be related to symptoms of fatigue.[26] Renal 1-a hydroxylase is responsible for the conversion of 25-hydroxyvitamin D to the active 1,25-dihydroxyvitamin D (cholecalciferol), which in turn causes calcium absorption from the gut and regulates bone mineralization. In CKD, this terminal activation is adversely affected and leads to cholecalciferol and calcium deficiency. Secondary hyperparathyroidism occurs (in part due to hyperplasia of the parathyroid gland in the absence of upregulation of vitamin D receptors in the PTH cells) to correct this hypocalcemia.

Cachexia of Chronic Kidney Disease

Protein energy wasting (PEW) is common in advanced stages of CKD.[27,28] This is a condition in which there is loss of muscle and visceral protein stores, decreased weight and protein/energy intake, and abnormal biochemical indicators (elevated C-reactive protein and hypoalbuminemia).[29] It is associated with increased cardiovascular disease, infections, and death.[19,30–32] Poor nutritional status/PEW has also been implicated as a cause of fatigue in CKD.[8]

PEW is characterized by net protein catabolism. A proinflammatory state (abnormal tumor necrosis factor α [TNF-α] and interleukin-6, alteration in myostatin, insulinlike growth factor 1, suppressor of cytokine signaling 2 signaling), increased resting metabolic rate/energy expenditure in the face of inadequate calorie intake, and inefficient use of exogenous amino acids in muscle protein synthesis are thought to be the reasons behind the catabolism. Anorexia due to CKD-associated dysgeusia, impaired gastric motility, elevated cytokines, and abnormal appetite hormones (leptin and ghrelin), leads to decreased oral intake and exacerbates the state of malnutrition in CKD. Insulin resistance, in part attributable to Vitamin D deficiency in CKD, leading to a loss of lean body mass, also plays a contributory role in the development of PEW syndrome.[29,33]

Depression

A significant proportion of patients with CKD, especially those on dialysis, exhibit depressive symptoms.[2] Up to a quarter of patients with CKD have symptoms consistent with a diagnosis of depressive disorder based on DSM-IV criteria.[34] Depression, as well as being associated with a lack of energy and fatigue, has been linked with poor outcomes, such as increased rates of hospitalization, cardiovascular events, and mortality in patients with CKD.[35]

Treatment of Fatigue in CKD

There is no specific treatment for fatigue in CKD. Management strategies focus on targeting the previously mentioned factors involved in the pathogenesis of fatigue.

Therapy of anemia includes judicious use of erythropoiesis-simulating agents (ESA) and iron supplementation. Treatment generally starts once hemoglobin levels drop below 10 g/dL. The goal of therapy is to bring levels between 11 and 12 g/dL.[36] Recent data suggest that correction of anemia with use of ESAs results in amelioration of fatigue, especially in patients whose hemoglobin levels are lower than 10 g/dL.[3,37,38] Once the desired hemoglobin level is obtained, the dosage or frequency of ESAs can be reduced to prevent complications. Higher hemoglobin targets (>13 g/dL) with ESAs have been linked with adverse outcomes, such as cardiovascular events, increased rate of hospitalizations, and death.[39,40] Iron supplementation, oral or parenteral, aims to keep transferrin saturation between 20% and 50% and ferritin levels between 100 and 800 ng/mL. Periodic monitoring of both hemoglobin/hematocrit and iron studies are advised in more advanced stages of CKD. An anemia workup, including stool for occult blood, red cell indices, reticulocytes, and hematological consultation if necessary, should be performed on detection of low hemoglobin levels, before attributing it solely to anemia of CKD.[36]

Low-dose active oral vitamin D sterol supplementation is recommended in stage 3 CKD and beyond, depending on levels of 25-hydroxyvitamin D, calcium, phosphate, and intact PTH.[41] Vitamin D supplementation suppresses intact PTH concentration and has been shown to improve bone histologic changes and bone mineral density in patients with renal osteodystrophy associated with secondary hyperparathyroidism in CKD.[42–44] Vitamin D also has possible beneficial effect on mortality in CKD.[45] Therapy should be initiated when serum levels of 25(OH)-vitamin D are higher than 30 ng/mL (75 nmol/L), and plasma levels of intact PTH are above the target range for the CKD stage (70 pmol/L for stage 3 and 110 pmol/L for stage 4 and 5), and corrected total calcium and serum phosphorus levels are less than 9.5 mg/dL and less than 4.6 mg/dL respectively. Supplementation should be avoided in patients with rapidly worsening renal function or who are not compliant with medications or follow-up. Careful monitoring of intact PTH, calcium, and phosphorus levels is recommended for patients on vitamin D with reduction in doses if levels exceed recommended thresholds. Dietary phosphate restriction, phosphate binders, and, if required, parathyroidectomy (for severe hyperparathyroidism refractory to medical therapy) can be used as adjunctive treatment.[41]

Management of wasting/malnutrition in CKD is difficult. Nutritional supplementation and correction of acidosis, with use of oral alkalis or higher dialysate lactate concentration, provides modest benefit in nutritional status.[29] Work is under way to assess efficacy of various approaches, such as appetite stimulants, ghrelin agonists, growth hormone use, leptin signal modulation, and ubiquitin-proteasome inhibitors.

Management of depression in CKD poses a special challenge. Unfortunately, the safety profile and effectiveness of antidepressants has not been well established in chronic renal disease; most trials on antidepressants excluded patients with CKD. Concerns about drug interactions, half-life and elimination (especially in patients on hemodialysis), and side effects abound. Caution should be exercised when using antidepressants in CKD. Nonpharmacologic measures, such as cognitive behavior therapy, exercise programs, changes in dialysis regimen (more frequent sessions), can be useful.[34,35]

SLEEPINESS IN RENAL DISEASE

Sleep disturbances are commonly encountered in renal disease, especially dialysis-dependent stage 5 CKD.[2,46] Insomnia is the most common sleep abnormality reported by patients with renal disorders. Daytime sleepiness can also be present, although reported rates vary across studies.[8,47] Similar to fatigue, there is no specific treatment for somnolence other than management of underlying renal disorder and supportive care. Adequate sleep hygiene measures (including adequate allocated duration for nocturnal sleep, comfortable sleeping environment, avoidance of stimulants, such as caffeine and nicotine close to bedtime, and so forth) should be adopted. Somnolence encountered in the setting of severe uremia/metabolic encephalopathy of renal disease requires initiation of dialysis.

Key Points

- Fatigue is a feature of both acute and chronic renal disease.
- Pathophysiology of fatigue in CKD includes uremic milieu, anemia of CKD, depression, protein energy wasting, and renal mineral and bone disorder.

- Treatment focuses on correction of anemia with ESAs and iron supplementation, vitamin D supplementation and phosphate binders, nutritional supplements and correction of acidosis, and cautious use of antidepressants.

ENDOCRINE DISORDERS

Various endocrine disorders may manifest themselves through fatigue or sleep disturbances. Some of the common endocrine abnormalities associated with these manifestations are discussed in this section.

THYROID

Screening for thyroid dysfunction should be considered in all patients suspected of sleep disorders. In hypothyroidism (underactive thyroid function), patients are symptomatic with fatigue, mental sluggishness, and increased somnolence.[48] Other symptoms include weight gain, cold intolerance, dry skin, hair loss, edema, and constipation. Coma can occur in severe cases. Treatment is targeted toward normalization of thyroid hormone levels with levothyroxine replacement. Periodic thyroid stimulating hormone measurements are used as a guiding tool to assess adequacy of dose.

On the other end of the spectrum, in hyperthyroidism (overactive thyroid state), a disruptive sleep pattern, insomnia, and multiple awakenings may be present. Increased resting metabolism occurs in thyrotoxicosis; often patients complain of palpitations keeping them up at night. Other clinical manifestations include weight loss, heat intolerance, tremors, tachycardia, and diarrhea. Specific treatment is based on the etiology of thyrotoxicosis with the ultimate aim of normalizing the levothyroxine levels. The commonest cause of hyperthyroidism is Grave disease; other etiologies include toxic multinodular goiter, autonomously functioning toxic thyroid nodule, and some rare conditions, eg, Struma ovarii.[49] Treatment options consist of thionamides, I-131 ablation, and surgery.

In addition to direct hormonal effects, sleep disorders can occur due to mechanical complications arising from thyroid disease. For example, obstruction caused by an enlarged thyroid or multinodular goiter can cause obstructive sleep apnea.[50] Complications from thyroid surgery can also contribute to obstruction and breathing abnormalities resulting in sleep disordered breathing.

PITUITARY, GONADAL, AND ADRENAL AXIS

Adrenal insufficiency, either primary or secondary (from pituitary failure), classically causes fatigue, lethargy, and sleepiness.[51] This serious disorder can be life threatening if left untreated. Other clinical manifestations include weight loss, hypotension, hyponatremia, gastrointestinal symptoms, and changes in pigmentation. Assessment of pituitary and adrenal axis hormones should be performed in patients with the these symptoms; 8 AM serum or salivary cortisol and electrolytes, followed by corticotrophin-stimulation testing, and further evaluation by an endocrinologist should be considered. Fatigue and sleep disruption generally resolves once appropriate treatment with steroid replacement is commenced. Therapy needs to be monitored closely to avoid steroid-induced side effects (eg, Cushing syndrome).

Pituitary insufficiency can result in multiple hormonal deficiencies: secondary adrenal failure, secondary hypothyroidism, growth hormone deficiency, secondary hypogonadism, and diabetes insipidus (DI).[52] Fatigue and sleep disturbances occur with most of these hormonal abnormalities.[52–54] In DI, polyuria, nocturia, and polydipsia can be significant and disruptive to a full night's sleep. Treatment with desmopressin is often timed at bedtime to minimize nocturia with a secondary benefit on sleep continuity.[55]

Hypogonadism can be primary or secondary to various causes, including genetic, metabolic, infectious, and autoimmune conditions. It results in multiple nonspecific symptoms. Low energy can be seen in both hypogonadal men and women. A detailed workup to assess the etiology as well as consideration of treatment of risk factors is important before hormone replacement is initiated.[48]

Low testosterone levels deserve a separate mention, as these may often occur secondary to sleep disorders, with sleep apnea being a well-documented cause of central hypogonadism.[56,57] Any patient identified to have low testosterone levels with untreated sleep disorders should not be started on testosterone replacement empirically. In most cases, the deficiency will resolve once the sleep apnea is optimally treated.[58]

DIABETES MELLITUS

Diabetes mellitus per se does not result in disturbed sleep; however, sleep disruption can occur from symptoms attributable to poor diabetes control. In patients with hyperglycemia, nocturia and polydipsia cause multiple nocturnal awakenings. Conversely, hypoglycemia (from insulin and oral hypoglycemic medications), may result in a deep sleep, especially in patients who have hypoglycemia unawareness. "Hypoglycemic coma" can occur when the drop in blood sugars is severe enough. When awareness is still present,

the patient wakes up with hypoglycemic symptoms: sweating, pale, nauseous, and feeling weak. If this happens frequently, many patients become fearful of slipping into a coma and actually set up their alarms so they can wake up multiple times at night to check their blood glucose levels. With optimal management, the goal is to avoid overnight hypoglycemia completely. A change in the diabetic medications and/or diet pattern may be required to achieve this.[48]

CALCIUM DISORDERS

Hypercalcemia can result in fatigue, confusion, and even loss of consciousness if severe enough. Besides these neurologic manifestations, a high blood calcium level can cause polyuria, nocturia, and polydipsia, with or without nephrogenic diabetes insipidus; nausea, bone pain, and peptic ulcer disease can also occur with hypercalcemia. All of these can result in sleep initiation and maintenance insomnia. Assessment for calcium disorders and their treatment is necessary; correction of blood calcium levels will often correct these symptoms rapidly.[48]

PARATHYROID DISORDERS

The parathyroid glands, located in the neck, behind the thyroid, produce PTH. PTH, along with vitamin D, is the chief regulator of calcium homeostasis in humans. It increases serum calcium concentration by enhancing bone resorption, increasing renal reabsorption of calcium, and stimulating synthesis of 1,25-dihydroxyvitamin D that in turn stimulates gastrointestinal calcium absorption. Calcium and vitamin D inhibit PTH synthesis and release.[1]

Abnormalities in parathyroid function lead to deranged calcium homeostasis. Signs and symptoms of parathyroid disease are predominantly a function of abnormal calcium levels. Fatigue is commonly seen with hypercalcemia, but can also be present with hypocalcemia.[26] It is a nonspecific symptom; other manifestations serve as clues to disturbed calcium levels being the reason behind the fatigue. Paresthesias, perioral numbness, tetany, and positive Chvostek and Trousseau signs are seen with hypocalcemia. Polyuria, polydipsia, dehydration, constipation, nausea, vomiting, muscle weakness, impaired concentration, lethargy, and altered mental status are clues toward the presence of hypercalcemia. Sleepiness, unless in the setting of early stupor with severe hypercalcemia, is generally not seen in parathyroid disorders.

Once the diagnosis of hypocalcemia or hypercalcemia is confirmed, the workup should include assessment for parathyroid disease. Management is according to the underlying etiology. Hypocalcemia attributable to hypoparathyroidism is generally treated with medications. Hypoparathyroidism can be idiopathic, hereditary, or secondary to trauma or surgery in the neck. Treatment includes calcium and vitamin D supplementation.[59] Careful monitoring of calcium, phosphate, and creatinine levels is required to avoid potential vitamin D intoxication; and thiazide diuretics to counter calciuria induced by vitamin D and calcium supplementation.

Hyperparathyroidism resulting in hypercalcemia is generally due to parathyroid adenomas or hyperplasia. Surgical resection is the definitive therapy, especially in the setting of declining renal function or bone disease. However, medical management (bisphosphonates, cincacalcet, estrogen replacement therapy, hydration, and exercise) can be useful in early disease and in patients who are not good operative candidates.[60]

Key Points

- Fatigue is a nonspecific symptom accompanying almost all endocrine abnormalities.
- Thyroid, pituitary, adrenal, gonadal, and parathyroid disorders are diagnosed by measurement of serum hormone levels.
- Treatment depends on etiology and includes both medical and surgical options. The underlying principle is normalization of serum hormone levels.

HEMATOLOGICAL DISORDERS

This section covers fatigue associated with anemia and other hematological conditions.

Anemia

Anemia is a highly prevalent condition that not only results in a considerable economic burden but also adversely affects the patient's quality of life (**Fig. 1**).[61] Unfortunately, it remains underrecognized and, therefore, undertreated in most cases. There are many causes of anemia: they are broadly categorized as acute or chronic. Acute anemia is generally seen in the setting of acute blood loss or hemolysis and generally presents with dyspnea or dizziness; fatigue is not a common symptom.

The present review focuses on chronic anemia. This frequently occurs because of an underlying medical condition, nutritional deficiency, or aging. It is a very common cause of fatigue. Correction of the underlying anemia usually results in improvement of health and quality of life of the affected individual.

Definition and epidemiology of anemia

Anemia has been defined by the World Health Organization as a hemoglobin level below 13.5 g/dL in males and postmenopausal females, and lower than 12 g/dL in premenopausal females. There has been a lot of controversy regarding this arbitrary definition that has been further challenged by the data from the National Health and Nutrition Examination Survey III study.[62] The findings of this study suggest that the lower limits of hemoglobin for anemia should vary with age, sex, and race. The study also proposed that values as low as 12.7 g/dL for black men older than 60 years and 11.5 g/dL for black women older than 20 years are appropriate.[63] Another important limitation to recognize is that the "normal" range will vary in patients living in high altitudes[64] and among

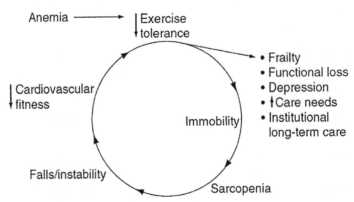

Fig. 1. The association of anemia with morbidity and fatigue. In this model, anemia causes reduced exercise tolerance, leading in turn to relative immobility, muscle wasting (sarcopenia), falls, and diminished cardiovascular fitness that further reduces exercise tolerance. This downward spiral produces the consequences listed on the right: frailty, dependency, and depression. (*From* Robinson B. Cost of anemia in the elderly. J Am Geriatr Soc 2003;51:S14–7; with permission.)

smokers,[65] athletes,[66] and patients with chronic diseases, such as malignancy, connective tissue disorder, or kidney or heart disease.[67]

Data from Center of Disease Control and Prevention indicate that about 5.3 million ambulatory care visits are a result of complaints related to a primary diagnosis of anemia and that chronic anemia is seen in 19% of all nursing home residents.[68] The estimated prevalence of anemia increases with age but varies widely. The main causes of chronic anemia are listed in **Table 2**. Anemia of chronic disease (AOCD) accounts for most of these cases.[69]

Pathophysiology of chronic anemia

Common causes of anemia, especially in the older age group, include nutritional deficiencies (iron, vitamin B12, and/or folic acid), anemia of chronic inflammation, and renal insufficiency. The postulated underlying mechanism for the latter 2 conditions is EPO deficiency. In CKD, this EPO deficiency is absolute, whereas in the case of AOCD, the EPO deficiency is relative. A combination of conditions resulting in anemia is quite common in the elderly.

The hallmark of AOCD is an inappropriate rise of serum erythropoietin levels with a decline of hemoglobin.[67] AOCD is primarily immune driven.

Proinflammatory cytokines, such as interferon γ, lipopolysaccharides, and TNF-α, cause a disturbance in iron homeostasis. This is characterized by increased uptake of iron by cells of the reticuloendothelial system with a subsequent decrease in transferrable iron available for effective erythropoiesis, resulting in anemia.[70] Lipopolysaccharides and interleukin-6 induce expression of hepcidin, a 25–amino acid protein, by the liver. Hepcidin acts as an iron-regulated acute-phase reactant. Once stimulated, it inhibits ferroprotein in the reticuloendothelial cells and gut enterocytes, thereby decreasing iron absorption and transport. Hepcidin is now known to play a major role in the pathogenesis of AOCD.[71] Moreover, inflammatory cytokines also cause impairment in the proliferation and differentiation of the erythroid precursors and increase their apoptosis. This is likely due to immune-mediated induction of apoptosis and direct toxic effects of the free radicals generated by the surrounding reticuloendothelial cells.[72]

EPO is a hormone produced by the kidneys and its expression is inversely proportional to the degree of tissue oxygenation and hemoglobin levels. In AOCD, cytokines cause blunting of the EPO response to the degree of anemia. In addition, these cytokines also result in downregulation of the EPO receptors on the erythroid precursors, further propagating impaired red cell production and anemia.[73] Finally, increased erythrophagocytosis during inflammation, along with direct damage to red blood cells by cytokines and free radicals, leads to a decreased erythrocyte half-life.[74]

Clinical consequences of chronic anemia

Anemia results in impaired oxygen delivery to the tissues, requiring a compensatory increase in cardiac output to maintain adequate tissue oxygenation. The increased cardiac output can result in high output cardiac failure with its accompanying manifestations, including fatigue. In patients with known congestive heart failure, anemia has been shown to increase rehospitalization rates and mortality.[75,76]

The more severe consequences of anemia are seen in the elderly. In this age group, anemia can cause decreased exercise tolerance, frailty, fatigue, and an overall worsening of performance status. In a prospective study of 1146 patients aged 71 and older, hemoglobin lower than 12 g/dL in women and 13 g/dL in men was determined to be an independent risk factor for physical decline in 4 years. The association of anemia and worsening performance status was seen even in patients who did not have a chronic illness (eg, malignancy, chronic kidney disease, diabetes).[77]

Table 2 Conditions associated with anemia of chronic disease	
Infections	Viral Bacterial Fungal Parasitic
Malignancy	Solid organ Hematological
Benign hematological disorders	Aplastic anemia, pure red aplasia, myelodysplasia Hemoglobinopathies Nutritional anemia Enzymopathies
Autoimmune	Systemic lupus erythematosus Rheumatoid arthritis Vasculitis Sarcoidosis Inflammatory bowel disease
Endocrine disorders	Hypothyroidism Hypogonadism
Chronic kidney disease	
Chronic rejection post solid organ transplantation	

Anemia increases the risk for falls, muscle wasting, and immobility in the elderly[78] and can lead to worsening of depression and dementia and increase in rehospitalization rates.[79] The Women Health and Aging study showed an increased risk of mortality in older women with hemoglobin levels lower than 13.4 g/dL.[80]

Anemia is also associated with an increased risk of complications and inferior outcome in a wide range of diseases and medical conditions. In pregnancy, anemia can result in preterm labor and low birth weight. In surgical patients, anemia significantly correlates with mortality, morbidity, and length of hospital stay.[81,82] It has also been well demonstrated that anemia in the postoperative and recovery period causes significant fatigue and adversely effects the quality of life.[83]

Cancer and Hematological Malignancies

Cancer, including both hematological and solid organ malignancies, is associated with fatigue in the vast majority of cases.[84,85] In a household survey of patients with cancer complaining of fatigue, 90% reported that it prevented them from living their normal life. In about 88% of the patients, alteration in their activities of daily living was attributed to fatigue, thus severely affecting their quality of life.[85]

Cancer-related fatigue is multifactorial. It encompasses a cluster of conditions that, along with the underlying disease, contribute to the development of fatigue. Among these are anemia, depression, cachexia, sleep deprivation, and the effect of treatment, such as chemotherapy and radiation.

Anemia is very common in patients with cancer[86,87] and appears to have an additive effect on fatigue and quality of life in addition to symptoms related to the cancer itself. In a recent survey, 2369 patients with cancer and anemia, 113 patients with cancer who did not have anemia, and 1010 individuals in the general US population were assessed for fatigue. Fatigue scores of the patients with cancer and anemia (at both baseline and on completion of anemia therapy) were significantly worse compared with the scores of patients with cancer who were not anemic, who, in turn, were worse compared with the scores of the general US population ($P<.001$). Within the group of patients with cancer and anemia, the degree of anemia (mild, moderate, or severe) itself was also predictive of the degree of fatigue ($P<.001$).[88]

The etiology of anemia in cancer can be a result of treatment or could be secondary to the disease itself. For example, hematological disorders, such as leukemia and multiple myeloma, universally cause anemia as a result of bone marrow replacement by neoplastic cells. In addition, proinflammatory cytokines produced by the malignancy inhibit erythropoiesis, resulting in anemia and fatigue.[89] Chemotherapy-induced anemia can be a result of impaired hematopoiesis, especially with cytotoxic drugs. In addition, certain drugs, such as platinum salts, can cause nephrotoxicity, which can lead to persistent anemia because of decreased production of EPO.[90]

Cancer chemotherapy and/or cytokines produced by the disease itself can also alter membrane transport in the erythrocytes resulting in changes in potassium, chloride, and magnesium ion fluxes. It has been postulated that erythrocyte magnesium levels may play a role in chronic fatigue syndrome in patients with cancer.[91]

Treatment

The rationale for the treatment of anemia is based on 2 principles. First, anemia can generally be deleterious in itself, resulting in dysfunction of vital structures, such as the heart. It can also adversely affect quality of life, because of fatigue and a decreased exercise tolerance. Second, anemia is associated with a poorer prognosis in a variety of conditions with increased risk of hospitalization and mortality, as mentioned previously. Thus, even moderate anemia warrants correction, especially in the elderly and/or those with additional comorbidities (such as coronary artery disease, pulmonary disease, or chronic kidney disease).[92] It has been shown that correction of anemia up to hemoglobin levels of 12 g/dL is associated with an improvement in the quality of life in patients with renal failure who are receiving dialysis and in patients with cancer who are undergoing chemotherapy.[93,94]

Correction of the underlying cause

It is important to assess for the underlying cause of anemia. Replenishment of nutrients in the case of vitamin B12, folic acid, and/or iron deficiency will lead to improvement of anemia and amelioration of symptoms of fatigue. Management of concomitant hypothyroidism or renal disease, both of which can contribute to anemia, is indicated if present. In cases in which no correctable cause can be identified, options include transfusion and ESAs.

Transfusions

Packed red blood cell transfusion is a quick and highly effective way to ameliorate symptoms of anemia. It has also been shown to improve clinical outcomes in certain settings. Blood transfusions have been shown to be beneficial in patients with myocardial infarction, with lower 30-day mortality with maintenance of hematocrit levels between 31% and 33% by blood transfusions.

However, blood transfusions should always be done cautiously. Studies have shown that although transfusions can help alleviate fatigue, their effect is usually transient and can increase mortality after 2 weeks.[95] A higher risk of postoperative mortality, pulmonary, and infectious complications is seen with intraoperative blood transfusion.[96] Other potential complications of transfusion therapy include risk of transfusion reactions, including severe reaction leading to multisystem organ failure, transmission of infections from improperly screened blood products, iron overload, and HLA alloimmunization. As a result of these deleterious consequences, existing guidelines for the management of anemia of chronic disease in patients with cancer or CKD do not recommend long-term blood transfusion therapy.[95]

ESAs

ESAs are currently indicated for treatment of anemia in patients with CKD, to lessen their need for chronic transfusion support. There are 2 types of ESA products available in the market: erythropoietin alpha and darbopoietin alpha. These 2 products differ in terms of their pharmacologic compound modifications, receptor-binding affinity, and serum half-life, thus allowing for alternative dosing and scheduling strategies. ESAs are also useful in cancer-related anemia. A recent meta-analysis suggested that a rise in hemoglobin by 2 g/dL, with the use of ESAs, resulted in meaningful improvements in fatigue, which, in turn, was associated with improved physical, functional, emotional, and overall well-being.[97]

Although the positive short-term beneficial effects of ESAs, such as improvement of fatigue and reduced need for blood transfusions have been well documented, long-term analysis of earlier studies now reveals that ESAs can have serious late toxicities. A meta-analysis of 13,933 patients with cancer from 53 trials reported an increased mortality and worsened overall survival in the patients receiving either one of the ESAs.[98] The results of this meta-analysis and several other studies have led to recommendations by American Society of Oncology and American Society of Hematology that urge extreme caution with the use of ESAs in patients with cancer.[98,99] If used, ESAs should be administered at the lowest possible dose to achieve the minimum hemoglobin level at which transfusions can be avoided.[100]

Key Points

- Anemia is the most common hematological condition associated with fatigue and is

associated with significant morbidity and mortality. It is also the primary mechanism of fatigue for most hematological disorders, including malignancies, such as leukemia and lymphomas.
- Cytokines and a proinflammatory state seen in anemia of chronic disease and in cancers can contribute to fatigue.
- Therapy for hematological conditions (such as chemotherapy for leukemias) can itself cause fatigue.
- Treatment focuses on correction of the underlying cause of the fatigue. Judicious use of ESAs and blood products may be required.

SLEEP DISORDERS ASSOCIATED WITH MEDICAL CONDITIONS

Some sleep disorders are more prevalent in certain medical conditions. Obstructive sleep apnea is more common in patients with hypothyroidism and acromegaly because of changes in upper airway anatomy that can take place with these diseases.[101] Periodic breathing of sleep/central sleep apnea can occur in patients with chronic kidney disease.[102–104] Restless legs syndrome has been linked with anemia and chronic renal disease, whereas sleep-related leg cramps are common with fluid and electrolyte imbalance seen with renal and metabolic disorders.[102,103,105,106] When evaluating sleepiness and fatigue in endocrine, renal, and hematological diseases, it is important to assess for specific sleep disorders associated with these conditions. If such sleep disorders are present, they need to be treated as per usual recommendations.

SUMMARY

Fatigue is a protective mechanism that aids in recovery from physical and mental stress in healthy individuals. In the setting of medical disorders, however, it can be severely debilitating and can have significant consequences. A number of diseases can be associated with fatigue. Included among these are CKD, endocrine disorders, anemia, and other hematological conditions. There is no specific treatment of fatigue linked to these medical conditions. Therapeutic strategies focus on treatment of the underlying medical illness.

REFERENCES

1. Cecil RL, Goldman L, Schafer AI. Goldman's Cecil Medicine. 24th edition. Philadelphia: Elsevier/Saunders; 2012.
2. Murtagh FE, Addington-Hall J, Higginson IJ. The prevalence of symptoms in end-stage renal

disease: a systematic review. Adv Chronic Kidney Dis 2007;14:82–99.

3. Johansen KL, Finkelstein FO, Revicki DA, et al. Systematic review of the impact of erythropoiesis-stimulating agents on fatigue in dialysis patients. Nephrol Dial Transplant 2012;27(6):2418–25.

4. Fatigue in CKD. Nephrol News Issues 2004;18:S1–8.

5. Jhamb M, Pike F, Ramer S, et al. Impact of fatigue on outcomes in the hemodialysis (HEMO) study. Am J Nephrol 2011;33:515–23.

6. Koyama H, Fukuda S, Shoji T, et al. Fatigue is a predictor for cardiovascular outcomes in patients undergoing hemodialysis. Clin J Am Soc Nephrol 2010;5:659–66.

7. National Kidney Foundation. K/DOQI clinical practice guidelines for chronic kidney disease: evaluation, classification, and stratification. Am J Kidney Dis 2002;39:S1–266.

8. Karakan S, Sezer S, Ozdemir FN. Factors related to fatigue and subgroups of fatigue in patients with end-stage renal disease. Clin Nephrol 2011;76:358–64.

9. Astor BC, Muntner P, Levin A, et al. Association of kidney function with anemia: the Third National Health and Nutrition Examination Survey (1988-1994). Arch Intern Med 2002;162:1401–8.

10. McClellan W, Aronoff SL, Bolton WK, et al. The prevalence of anemia in patients with chronic kidney disease. Curr Med Res Opin 2004;20:1501–10.

11. Ratcliffe PJ. Molecular biology of erythropoietin. Kidney Int 1993;44:887–904.

12. Thomas R, Kanso A, Sedor JR. Chronic kidney disease and its complications. Prim Care 2008;35:329–44, vii.

13. Nurko S. Anemia in chronic kidney disease: causes, diagnosis, treatment. Cleve Clin J Med 2006;73:289–97.

14. Chateauvieux S, Grigorakaki C, Morceau F, et al. Erythropoietin, erythropoiesis and beyond. Biochem Pharmacol 2011;82:1291–303.

15. McPherson RJ, Juul SE. Recent trends in erythropoietin-mediated neuroprotection. Int J Dev Neurosci 2008;26:103–11.

16. Calapai G, Marciano MC, Corica F, et al. Erythropoietin protects against brain ischemic injury by inhibition of nitric oxide formation. Eur J Pharmacol 2000;401:349–56.

17. Catania MA, Marciano MC, Parisi A, et al. Erythropoietin prevents cognition impairment induced by transient brain ischemia in gerbils. Eur J Pharmacol 2002;437:147–50.

18. Hsu CY, McCulloch CE, Curhan GC. Epidemiology of anemia associated with chronic renal insufficiency among adults in the United States: results from the Third National Health and Nutrition Examination Survey. J Am Soc Nephrol 2002;13:504–10.

19. Kalantar-Zadeh K, Block G, McAllister CJ, et al. Appetite and inflammation, nutrition, anemia, and clinical outcome in hemodialysis patients. Am J Clin Nutr 2004;80:299–307.

20. Kestenbaum B, Sampson JN, Rudser KD, et al. Serum phosphate levels and mortality risk among people with chronic kidney disease. J Am Soc Nephrol 2005;16:520–8.

21. Stevens LA, Djurdjev O, Cardew S, et al. Calcium, phosphate, and parathyroid hormone levels in combination and as a function of dialysis duration predict mortality: evidence for the complexity of the association between mineral metabolism and outcomes. J Am Soc Nephrol 2004;15:770–9.

22. Young EW, Akiba T, Albert JM, et al. Magnitude and impact of abnormal mineral metabolism in hemodialysis patients in the Dialysis Outcomes and Practice Patterns Study (DOPPS). Am J Kidney Dis 2004;44:34–8.

23. Mejia N, Roman-Garcia P, Miar AB, et al. Chronic kidney disease—mineral and bone disorder: a complex scenario. Nefrologia 2011;31:514–9.

24. Slatopolsky E, Robson AM, Elkan I, et al. Control of phosphate excretion in uremic man. J Clin Invest 1968;47:1865–74.

25. Levin A, Bakris GL, Molitch M, et al. Prevalence of abnormal serum vitamin D, PTH, calcium, and phosphorus in patients with chronic kidney disease: results of the study to evaluate early kidney disease. Kidney Int 2007;71:31–8.

26. Oudesluys-Murphy AM, de Vries AC. Fatigue due to hypocalcaemia. Lancet 2002;359:443.

27. Kopple JD. McCollum Award Lecture, 1996: protein-energy malnutrition in maintenance dialysis patients. Am J Clin Nutr 1997;65:1544–57.

28. Kalantar-Zadeh K, Ikizler TA, Block G, et al. Malnutrition-inflammation complex syndrome in dialysis patients: causes and consequences. Am J Kidney Dis 2003;42:864–81.

29. Mak RH, Ikizler AT, Kovesdy CP, et al. Wasting in chronic kidney disease. J Cachexia Sarcopenia Muscle 2011;2:9–25.

30. Rambod M, Bross R, Zitterkoph J, et al. Association of Malnutrition-Inflammation Score with quality of life and mortality in hemodialysis patients: a 5-year prospective cohort study. Am J Kidney Dis 2009;53:298–309.

31. Pupim LB, Caglar K, Hakim RM, et al. Uremic malnutrition is a predictor of death independent of inflammatory status. Kidney Int 2004;66:2054–60.

32. Bonanni A, Mannucci I, Verzola D, et al. Protein-energy wasting and mortality in chronic kidney disease. Int J Environ Res Public Health 2011;8:1631–54.

33. Meuwese CL, Carrero JJ, Stenvinkel P. Recent insights in inflammation-associated wasting in patients with chronic kidney disease. Contrib Nephrol 2011;171:120–6.

34. Finkelstein FO, Wuerth D, Finkelstein SH. An approach to addressing depression in patients with chronic kidney disease. Blood Purif 2010;29: 121–4.

35. Hedayati SS, Finkelstein FO. Epidemiology, diagnosis, and management of depression in patients with CKD. Am J Kidney Dis 2009;54:741–52.

36. KDOQI, National Kidney Foundation. KDOQI clinical practice guidelines and clinical practice recommendations for anemia in chronic kidney disease. Am J Kidney Dis 2006;47:S11–145.

37. Pfeffer MA, Burdmann EA, Chen CY, et al. A trial of darbepoetin alfa in type 2 diabetes and chronic kidney disease. N Engl J Med 2009;361:2019–32.

38. Gandra SR, Finkelstein FO, Bennett AV, et al. Impact of erythropoiesis-stimulating agents on energy and physical function in nondialysis CKD patients with anemia: a systematic review. Am J Kidney Dis 2010;55:519–34.

39. Singh AK, Szczech L, Tang KL, et al. Correction of anemia with epoetin alfa in chronic kidney disease. N Engl J Med 2006;355:2085–98.

40. Drueke TB, Locatelli F, Clyne N, et al. Normalization of hemoglobin level in patients with chronic kidney disease and anemia. N Engl J Med 2006;355: 2071–84.

41. National Kidney Foundation. K/DOQI clinical practice guidelines for bone metabolism and disease in chronic kidney disease. Am J Kidney Dis 2003;42: S1–201.

42. Nordal KP, Dahl E, Halse J, et al. Long-term low-dose calcitriol treatment in predialysis chronic renal failure: can it prevent hyperparathyroid bone disease? Nephrol Dial Transplant 1995;10: 203–6.

43. Cannella G, Bonucci E, Rolla D, et al. Evidence of healing of secondary hyperparathyroidism in chronically hemodialyzed uremic patients treated with long-term intravenous calcitriol. Kidney Int 1994;46:1124–32.

44. Andress DL, Norris KC, Coburn JW, et al. Intravenous calcitriol in the treatment of refractory osteitis fibrosa of chronic renal failure. N Engl J Med 1989; 321:274–9.

45. Kovesdy CP, Ahmadzadeh S, Anderson JE, et al. Association of activated vitamin D treatment and mortality in chronic kidney disease. Arch Intern Med 2008;168:397–403.

46. Davis ID, Greenbaum LA, Gipson D, et al. Prevalence of sleep disturbances in children and adolescents with chronic kidney disease. Pediatr Nephrol 2012;27:451–9.

47. Roumelioti ME, Wentz A, Schneider MF, et al. Sleep and fatigue symptoms in children and adolescents with CKD: a cross-sectional analysis from the chronic kidney disease in children (CKiD) study. Am J Kidney Dis 2010;55:269–80.

48. Gardner DG, Greenspan FS, Shoback DM. Greenspan's basic & clinical endocrinology. 9th edition. New York: McGraw-Hill Medical; 2011.

49. Trzepacz PT, Klein I, Roberts M, et al. Graves' disease: an analysis of thyroid hormone levels and hyperthyroid signs and symptoms. Am J Med 1989; 87:558–61.

50. Gutierrez T, Leong AC, Pang L, et al. Multinodular thyroid goitre causing obstructive sleep apnoea syndrome. J Laryngol Otol 2012;126:190–5.

51. Oelkers W. Adrenal insufficiency. N Engl J Med 1996;335:1206–12.

52. Vance ML. Hypopituitarism. N Engl J Med 1994; 330:1651–62.

53. Copinschi G, Nedeltcheva A, Leproult R, et al. Sleep disturbances, daytime sleepiness, and quality of life in adults with growth hormone deficiency. J Clin Endocrinol Metab 2010;95:2195–202.

54. Pinsky MR, Hellstrom WJ. Hypogonadism, ADAM, and hormone replacement. Ther Adv Urol 2010;2: 99–104.

55. Vande Walle J, Stockner M, Raes A, et al. Desmopressin 30 years in clinical use: a safety review. Curr Drug Saf 2007;2:232–8.

56. Santamaria JD, Prior JC, Fleetham JA. Reversible reproductive dysfunction in men with obstructive sleep apnoea. Clin Endocrinol (Oxf) 1988;28: 461–70.

57. Luboshitzky R, Aviv A, Hefetz A, et al. Decreased pituitary-gonadal secretion in men with obstructive sleep apnea. J Clin Endocrinol Metab 2002;87: 3394–8.

58. Grunstein RR, Handelsman DJ, Lawrence SJ, et al. Neuroendocrine dysfunction in sleep apnea: reversal by continuous positive airways pressure therapy. J Clin Endocrinol Metab 1989;68:352–8.

59. Shoback D. Clinical practice. Hypoparathyroidism. N Engl J Med 2008;359:391–403.

60. Marcocci C, Cetani F. Clinical practice. Primary hyperparathyroidism. N Engl J Med 2011;365: 2389–97.

61. Nissenson AR, Wade S, Goodnough T, et al. Economic burden of anemia in an insured population. J Manag Care Pharm 2005;11:565–74.

62. Beutler E, Waalen J. The definition of anemia: what is the lower limit of normal of the blood hemoglobin concentration? Blood 2006;107:1747–50.

63. Looker AC, Dallman PR, Carroll MD, et al. Prevalence of iron deficiency in the United States. JAMA 1997;277:973–6.

64. Ruiz-Arguelles GJ. Altitude above sea level as a variable for definition of anemia. Blood 2006;108: 2131 [author reply: 2].

65. Leifert JA. Anaemia and cigarette smoking. Int J Lab Hematol 2008;30:177–84.

66. Dufaux B, Hoederath A, Streitberger I, et al. Serum ferritin, transferrin, haptoglobin, and iron

in middle- and long-distance runners, elite rowers, and professional racing cyclists. Int J Sports Med 1981;2:43–6.

67. Cullis JO. Diagnosis and management of anaemia of chronic disease: current status. Br J Haematol 2011;154:289–300.

68. Schappert SM, Rechtsteiner EA. Ambulatory medical care utilization estimates for. Vital Health Stat 13 2007;(169):1–38.

69. Weiss G, Goodnough LT. Anemia of chronic disease. N Engl J Med 2005;352:1011–23.

70. Ludwiczek S, Aigner E, Theurl I, et al. Cytokine-mediated regulation of iron transport in human monocytic cells. Blood 2003;101:4148–54.

71. Rossi E. Hepcidin—the iron regulatory hormone. Clin Biochem Rev 2005;26:47–9.

72. Spivak JL. Iron and the anemia of chronic disease. Oncology (Williston Park) 2002;16:25–33.

73. Wang W, Zhang MH, Yu Y, et al. Influence of tumor necrosis factor-alpha and interferon-gamma on erythropoietin production and erythropoiesis in cancer patients with anemia. Zhonghua Xue Ye Xue Za Zhi 2007;28:681–4 [in Chinese].

74. Tracey KJ, Wei H, Manogue KR, et al. Cachectin/tumor necrosis factor induces cachexia, anemia, and inflammation. J Exp Med 1988;167:1211–27.

75. McMurray JJ. What are the clinical consequences of anemia in patients with chronic heart failure? J Card Fail 2004;10:S10–2.

76. Steinborn W, Doehner W, Anker SD. Anemia in chronic heart failure—frequency and prognostic impact. Clin Nephrol 2003;60(Suppl 1):S103–7.

77. Penninx BW, Guralnik JM, Onder G, et al. Anemia and decline in physical performance among older persons. Am J Med 2003;115:104–10.

78. Cesari M, Penninx BW, Pahor M, et al. Inflammatory markers and physical performance in older persons: the InCHIANTI study. J Gerontol A Biol Sci Med Sci 2004;59:242–8.

79. Santos IS, Scazufca M, Lotufo PA, et al. Anemia and dementia among the elderly: the Sao Paulo Ageing & Health Study. Int Psychogeriatr 2012; 24:74–81.

80. Chaves PH, Ashar B, Guralnik JM, et al. Looking at the relationship between hemoglobin concentration and prevalent mobility difficulty in older women. Should the criteria currently used to define anemia in older people be reevaluated? J Am Geriatr Soc 2002;50:1257–64.

81. Leichtle SW, Mouawad NJ, Lampman R, et al. Does preoperative anemia adversely affect colon and rectal surgery outcomes? J Am Coll Surg 2011; 212:187–94.

82. Dunne JR, Malone D, Tracy JK, et al. Perioperative anemia: an independent risk factor for infection, mortality, and resource utilization in surgery. J Surg Res 2002;102:237–44.

83. Conlon NP, Bale EP, Herbison GP, et al. Postoperative anemia and quality of life after primary hip arthroplasty in patients over 65 years old. Anesth Analg 2008;106:1056–61 [table of contents].

84. Portenoy RK, Thaler HT, Kornblith AB, et al. Symptom prevalence, characteristics and distress in a cancer population. Qual Life Res 1994;3:183–9.

85. Curt GA, Breitbart W, Cella D, et al. Impact of cancer-related fatigue on the lives of patients: new findings from the Fatigue Coalition. Oncologist 2000;5:353–60.

86. Birgegard G, Aapro MS, Bokemeyer C, et al. Cancer-related anemia: pathogenesis, prevalence and treatment. Oncology (Williston Park) 2005; 68(Suppl 1):3–11.

87. Barrett-Lee P, Bokemeyer C, Gascon P, et al. Management of cancer-related anemia in patients with breast or gynecologic cancer: new insights based on results from the European Cancer Anemia Survey. Oncologist 2005;10:743–57.

88. Cella D, Lai JS, Chang CH, et al. Fatigue in cancer patients compared with fatigue in the general United States population. Cancer 2002;94:528–38.

89. Dicato M, Plawny L, Diederich M. Anemia in cancer. Ann Oncol 2010;21(Suppl 7):vii167–72.

90. Rodgers GM 3rd, Becker PS, Bennett CL, et al. Cancer- and chemotherapy-induced anemia. J Natl Compr Canc Netw 2008;6:536–64.

91. Hinds G, Bell NP, McMaster D, et al. Normal red cell magnesium concentrations and magnesium loading tests in patients with chronic fatigue syndrome. Ann Clin Biochem 1994;31(Pt 5):459–61.

92. Murphy ST, Parfrey PS. The impact of anemia correction on cardiovascular disease in end-stage renal disease. Semin Nephrol 2000;20:350–5.

93. Moreno F, Sanz-Guajardo D, Lopez-Gomez JM, et al. Increasing the hematocrit has a beneficial effect on quality of life and is safe in selected hemodialysis patients. Spanish Cooperative Renal Patients Quality of Life Study Group of the Spanish Society of Nephrology. J Am Soc Nephrol 2000;11:335–42.

94. Littlewood TJ, Bajetta E, Nortier JW, et al. Epoetin Alfa Study Group. Effects of epoetin alfa on hematologic parameters and quality of life in cancer patients receiving nonplatinum chemotherapy: results of a randomized, double-blind, placebo-controlled trial. J Clin Oncol 2001;19:2865–74.

95. Preston NJ, Hurlow A, Brine J, et al. Blood transfusions for anaemia in patients with advanced cancer. Cochrane Database Syst Rev 2012;(2):CD009007.

96. O'Keeffe SD, Davenport DL, Minion DJ, et al. Blood transfusion is associated with increased morbidity and mortality after lower extremity revascularization. J Vasc Surg 2010;51:616–21, 621.e1–3.

97. Cella D, Kallich J, McDermott A, et al. The longitudinal relationship of hemoglobin, fatigue and quality of life in anemic cancer patients: results from

five randomized clinical trials. Ann Oncol 2004;15: 979–86.

98. Bohlius J, Schmidlin K, Brillant C, et al. Recombinant human erythropoiesis-stimulating agents and mortality in patients with cancer: a meta-analysis of randomised trials. Lancet 2009;373:1532–42.

99. Bennett CL, Silver SM, Djulbegovic B, et al. Venous thromboembolism and mortality associated with recombinant erythropoietin and darbepoetin administration for the treatment of cancer-associated anemia. JAMA 2008;299:914–24.

100. Rizzo JD, Brouwers M, Hurley P, et al. American Society of Clinical Oncology/American Society of Hematology clinical practice guideline update on the use of epoetin and darbepoetin in adult patients with cancer. J Clin Oncol 2010;28:4996–5010.

101. Attal P, Chanson P. Endocrine aspects of obstructive sleep apnea. J Clin Endocrinol Metab 2010; 95:483–95.

102. Kosmadakis GC, Medcalf JF. Sleep disorders in dialysis patients. Int J Artif Organs 2008;31:919–27.

103. American Academy of Sleep Medicine. The international classification of sleep disorders: diagnostic and coding manual. 2nd edition. Westchester (IL): American Academy of Sleep Medicine; 2005.

104. Langevin B, Fouque D, Leger P, et al. Sleep apnea syndrome and end-stage renal disease. Cure after renal transplantation. Chest 1993;103:1330–5.

105. Earley CJ. Clinical practice. Restless legs syndrome. N Engl J Med 2003;348:2103–9.

106. Monderer RS, Wu WP, Thorpy MJ. Nocturnal leg cramps. Curr Neurol Neurosci Rep 2010;10:53–9.

Universal Fatigue Management Strategies

Mary Rose, PsyD*, Nilgun Giray, MD

KEYWORDS

- Fatigue • Countermeasure • Sleep-deprived

KEY POINTS

- Type of fatigue or sleepiness is the first categorization needed before a management strategy can be used.
- Fatigue (rather than sleepiness) generated in the work place may be caused by not only overwork but by factors such as repetitive non-novel tasks leading to monotony, noise, and poorly lit environments.
- Individual factors and preferences must be incorporated into any sleepiness/fatigue management plan.
- Inadequate total sleep time and misalignment of circadian rhythm are the most significant contributors to disastrous human error in the work place.
- Pharmacologic and nonpharmacologic interventions to modify fatigue and sleepiness suggest some overall improvement in alertness and performance with a variety of agents.

Fatigue may have many origins. Research suggests that regardless of the cause, the symptoms may often be managed through similar strategies. As is discussed in other articles of this issue, most work-related fatigue is better classified as sleep deprivation and/or a misalignment of sleep schedule. Certainly, the first task at hand for identifying universal management strategies is to clarify what it is that is being managed. Categories and classifications of fatigue and sleepiness are discussed elsewhere in this article, although in general, differentiating sleepiness from mental and cognitive fatigue is an essential first step. Rarely is work-related fatigue of a physical nature in the modern work environment given the availability of mechanical equipment for such work; nonetheless, physical weariness is a common descriptor of fatigue even when physical labor is not present. Fatigue may be multifaceted; however, it is essential that all of the contributing causes be appropriately identified and addressed to avoid misattribution and use of inappropriate temporary strategies that may lead to a more serious lapse of attention,

as well as, a risk to health and safety. Likewise contributors to sleepiness need to be accurately identified.

The goals of this article are to (1) differentiate fatigue from sleepiness to define the precise goals of management, (2) identify and differentiate different broad causes of sleepiness and fatigue, and (3) identify universal strategies for managing both fatigue and sleepiness.

Fatigue (rather than sleepiness) generated in the work place may be caused not only by overwork, but also by factors such as repetitive nonnovel tasks leading to monotony, noise, and poorly lit environments. Although physical fatigue is problematic in some industries, strategies for managing physical fatigue would not follow the universal strategies the authors outline in this article. As nearly all attention in Occupational Medicine concerning fatigue is in fact focused on sleep, most of these strategies relate to maintaining alertness. Our consideration of fatigue and sleepiness management involves an array of strategies including pharmacologic, physiologic/behavioral, cognitive, and mechanical

Department of Medicine, Section of Pulmonary, Critical Care & Sleep Medicine, Baylor College of Medicine, Houston, TX 77025, USA
* Corresponding author.
E-mail address: MRosesleep@aol.com

Sleep Med Clin 8 (2013) 255–263
http://dx.doi.org/10.1016/j.jsmc.2013.02.004

strategies of management. These techniques are grossly broken into 2 major subsets: those that are preventative (used before the shift) and those that are operational (used during the shift).[1] One could further add that there are general strategies useful at all post-shift stages up to the time point immediately before the next shift. These strategies attempt to maximize productivity, reduce risk of injury, and decrease burnout. Occupational sleep medicine includes a vast array of professionals and duties. The professions of greatest research focus include jobs in the transportation, military, maritime, health care, mining, police, first responders, and energy industries. All of these jobs are essential to the functioning of an industrialized society and likewise, all carry a great weight with regard to safety and risk.

Hursh and Van Dogen[2] have reviewed biomathematical modeling of fatigue developed to predict performance changes in the workplace. They note that these typically are based upon 3 measures of sleep: homeostatic sleep-wake regulation, sleep inertia, and circadian variations in alertness and sleep propensity. Their model emphasizes sleep and circadian rhythm, rather than general weariness or fatigue as a focus of performance impairment. Belenky and Åkerstedt[3] note that across many fields an inappropriate model of using shift times, shift duration, and within shift breaks is often used with no regard to circadian rhythm or the role of increased homeostatic drive. One of the best examples of this is a common schedule developed by one of the major energy companies in which the worker has a 4-week cycle of 4 consecutive night shifts, followed by 3 days off duty, then works 3 consecutive day shifts, followed by 1 day off duty, works 3 consecutive night shifts, followed by 3 days off duty, work 4 consecutive day shift, then 7 consecutive days off duty. Despite the preponderance of evidence that such rotating schedules are detrimental to safety and health, they persist, presumably fueled some combination of financial pressure and administrative stagnancy against developing a more ergonomic and healthy model. However, the allure of a 7-day stint off duty likely garners favor by the employees as well. Workers will often report having become "used to" sleep loss and the public may assume that those who have professionally been working in a sleep-deprived or circadian misaligned schedule have somehow adjusted. This is largely a misperception. In our 24-hour society, that is not possible to completely forgo night shift work; we should consider both individual differences in ability to adjust to shift work and natural circadian factors that influence performance. Such an approach would facilitate our development of protocols to design universal strategies to combat fatigue and sleepiness and to identify which workers would

perform best (and most safely) with specific schedules. Some resilient workers may very well adjust to shift work and a reduced overall total sleep time below the norm (but only if this is consistent with their natural total sleep time).[4] However, many people greatly underestimate the amount of sleep that they require to function optimally. In a population study of more than 15,000 people, Ohayon found that 27.8% of adults reported excessive daytime sleepiness,[5] suggesting that in addition to wide underestimation of sleep need, a great many individuals suffer the consequences. With regard to a shift work and night shift model, it is notable that evening type students in one study were found to be more vulnerable to sleep loss, reported lower sleep quality, and higher work-related fatigue than did morning and intermediate type students,[6] suggesting that although evening type people may gravitate toward night shift work, they may be less suited to manage it biobehaviorally.

Type of fatigue or sleepiness is the first categorization needed before a management strategy can be used.

Fatigue may have multiple origins. Workers come to the workplace with the same medical conditions afflicting their lives outside of the work place. Any fatigue management program should offer screening (or at the very least education) for workers related to the common causes of fatigue and sleepiness. Education on differentiating between the 2 should also be provided. It would be helpful to screen for disorders such as insomnia, pain, obesity, diabetes, thyroid disease, depression, smoking, and iron deficiency. When such contributors are found for fatigue, the work place would benefit by ensuring that workers are adequately treated or their schedule is accommodated before returning to work, in lieu of simply masking fatigue through countermeasures. Some causes of fatigue have significant psychological and behavioral components that could easily benefit from education and at-work programs targeting identification and treatment.

At all 3 of the major time points (1) immediate pre-shift, (2) shift, and all (3) recovery Time points, training workers to identify their individual vulnerabilities and fatigue causes is essential. Not all workers with medical disorders commonly associated with fatigue will necessarily attribute the medical issues as the cause of *their* fatigue. One critical behavioral differentiation between sleepiness and fatigue is self-awareness and judgment. Those in sleep-deprived conditions have been shown to exhibit very poor self-judgment of their performance while sleep deprived. Also, many of us are vulnerable to overestimating our skills and level of safety when sleep deprived. This has been illuminated by several post-incidence disaster analyses. The effects of total and partial sleep loss have been associated with impaired judgment of deficit loss across a range of activities including driving simulation[7] and surgical skills.[8] This is extremely important as it suggests that regardless of the worker's self-assessment of need for strategies to offset sleepiness, such strategies should be *assumed* to be needed.

Aspects of fatiguing tasks or sleepiness that facilitate the importance of targeted manipulation include the complexity and type of work and the direness of loss of precision and skill with regard to impact on safety or risk. In some cases, even minor lapses in attention or judgment may lead to death of the worker or others. In such cases, even minor impairments need to be avoided. Such lapses of attention and/or of executive functioning may produce lethal outcomes when errors are made by emergency medical care workers, air traffic control controllers, pilots, truck drivers, and military combatants. By contrast there may be a less severe consequence of lapses in other types of work, for example assembly line workers or sales persons.

Different types of workers are prone to different vulnerabilities. Nearly all night shift workers and rotating shift workers experience circadian misalignment. Working nonregular daytime hours is associated with curtailed sleep, greater sleepiness, and more driving-related accidents.[9] Long haul drivers are most likely to experience overall sleep deprivation. Pilots may experience sleep deprivation, but may have some protection built into their task with presence of a co-pilot and strict regulation controlling flight hours. Additionally, with regard to cognitive fatigue, pilots have a broader array of instrument tasks needing frequent attention beyond that required of long haul drivers. This may minimize mental fatigue through increased need for task vigilance. Additionally, pilots typically are not alone in the cockpit. The presence of a co-pilot provides a safe guard against lapses of attention consequent to fatigue or sleepiness by either pilot, and may provide options for work rotation and breaks on prolonged flights.

Individual factors and preferences must be incorporated into any sleepiness/fatigue management plan. Factors that would play a role in this determination might include individual variables such as comorbid medical conditions, gender, age, medication sensitivities, and the individual's natural circadian rhythm (including morningness/eveningness). It is notable that insomnia, with its prevalence of 10%, that is worsened with shift work, is also likely to be at play with regard to both diminishing total sleep time (although those with insomnia often report very low daytime sleepiness), circadian misalignment, and in fueling fatigue in workers. Unfortunately, many with shift work sleep disorder (SWSD) are misdiagnosed by providers as having insomnia, given prescriptions for sleep aids and never educated about SWSD.

Screening for causes of sleepiness include obstructive sleep apnea, narcolepsy, elective sleep deprivation (which may include environmental factors such as family obligations, caring for another person at night, etc), and SWSD. Such screening serves to raise awareness, provide education, and to treat these common culprits. Individuals with obstructive sleep apnea and narcolepsy have greater risk for sleep-related auto accidents,[10,11] making these disorders particularly dangerous if untreated in a hazardous work place. Both sleep apnea and narcolepsy are easily diagnosed. Treatment of obstructive sleep apnea in particular is straight forward; however, therapeutic adherence to positive airway pressure treatment can be a challenge. Sleepiness, unlike fatigue, has a limited number of causes, and by definition, usually involves disruption or loss of sleep. Fatigue, however, has a greater number of possible causes that may stem from any combination of biologic, social, or psychological factors. Mental health disorders such as psychosis and the full gamut of mood disorders can include sleepiness and sleeplessness as symptoms. Hypersomnia and hyposomnia are symptoms rather than causes of mental disorders (although, as with most disorders, they may be greatly worsened by the presence of sleep disturbance).

Fatigue countermeasures need to recognize and tailor strategies to individual preferences. Although some techniques may be well supported overall for mitigating sleepiness and fatigue, they may be less optimal for specific workers due to side effects, medical comorbidity, strength of circadian drive, sensitivity, etc. The main universal strategies for managing fatigue and sleepiness include (1) acquiring adequate total sleep time, (2) proper circadian alignment, (3) strategic napping, (4) scheduled breaks (5) exercise (6) variation in work and introduction of novel tasks, (7) bright light exposure- particularly blue light (8) pharmacologic strategies, and (9) healthy eating habits. Techniques 1 to 3 are specific to managing sleepiness. Techniques 4 to 6 are specific to managing fatigue (although circadian misalignment may be associated with both sleepiness and fatigue). Techniques 7 to 9 may be beneficial in managing both fatigue and sleepiness. In addition to these, pharmacologic treatment such as caffeine-based, armodafinil-based, and amphetamine-based stimulants have been found to be effective for assuaging fatigue and sleepiness (**Table 1**). Although armodafinil is the only one that carries a

Table 1
Psychostimulants often used to mediate fatigue and sleepiness

Medication	Mechanism & Info	Class	Elimination 1/2 Life	Indications	Benefits	Risks
Modafinil (Provigil)	Mechanism of action uncertain & differs from other stimulants. Not a direct dopamine receptor agonist. Wakefulness promoted by modafinil may be attenuated by prazosin, an alpha 1-adrenergic antagonist.	IV Controlled	After multiple dosing is 15 h. It reaches steady state after 2–4 d.	Narcolepsy, shift-work sleep disorder, & residual sleepiness in airway managed OSA	Noncardiotoxic nonhabit forming	
Armodafinil (Nuvigil)	A nonamphetamine stimulant that enhances wakefulness. R enantiomer of modafinil	IV Controlled	15 h, steady state 7 d	Same as above	Noncardiotoxic nonhabit forming	
Caffeine	Adenosine receptor agonist	Not controlled	4.9–6 h. Wide variability between individuals	None approved	Readily available	Cardiotoxic tolerance
Amphetamines	Blocks reuptake of dopamine & NE in the presynaptic neuron, also release of NE & DA from presynaptic neuron into the synaptic space. L-amphetamine releases NE as well as dopamine.	II Controlled	10–14 h peak plasma 3 h	ADHD, narcolepsy, excessive daytime sleepiness	Powerful alerting properties	Cardiotoxic dependency

Drug	Mechanism	Schedule	Duration	Indication		
Adderall	Mixed amphetamine salts (dextroamphetamine saccharate & sulfate, amphetamine aspartate & sulfate)	II controlled	10 h	ADHD	Same for amphetamines	Same for amphetamines
Dexedrine (Dextroamphetamine)	Binds to presynaptic dopamine transporter, blocks dopamine re-uptake & causes dopamine release. Lower doses have preferential effect on attention, rather than motor activity	II Controlled	10–12 h	ADHD, narcolepsy	Same for amphetamines	Same for amphetamines
Vyvanse (Lisdexamfetamine dimesylate)	Prodrug of dextroamphetamine. After oral administration, lisdexamfetamine dimesylate is rapidly absorbed & converted to dextroamphetamine, which is responsible for the drug's activity	II Controlled	9.5 h	ADHD	Same for amphetamines	Same for amphetamines
Methylphenidate	Similar mechanism of action to dextroamphetamine, slower unset of action, but longer lasting	II Controlled		ADHD & narcolepsy		Cardiotoxic dependency
	Includes Ritalin, Concerta, Daytrana, Methylin					

Abbreviations: ADHD, attention-deficit hyperactivity disorder; DA, dopamine; NE, norepinephrine.

specific Food and Drug Administration–approved indication for shift work sleep disorder.

Inadequate total sleep time and misalignment of circadian rhythm are the most significant contributors to disastrous human error in the work place. Studies indicate that based upon large population studies, habitual restriction of total sleep time to less than 7 hours is associated with a significant increase to mortality rate.[12,13] The US National Transportation Safety Board has cited sleep loss as the cause for one-third of all fatal-to-driver traffic accidents as their probable cause. These accidents occur at higher speed and consequent to the lapse of attention, there is no attempt to correct course before the crash.[14] Investigation of numerous international disasters has also found that restricted total sleep time of the workers played a major role in decision-making surrounding disasters such as the Chernobyl nuclear meltdown, the Challenger explosion, the Bhopol chemical leak, and the Exxon Valdez oil spill.[15] In addition to the shift schedule itself, total sleep time is often reduced in shift workers consequent to prioritizing family activities and errands during daytime hours at the cost of sleep.

Workers in the transportation field often experience both sleep loss, misalignment of sleep, and mental fatigue. One comprehensive strategy to diminish accident-rates and errors due to fatigue and sleepiness involves limiting total work hours and requiring rest/nap periods. Research suggests that workers are more vulnerable to accidents between midnight and 6 AM,[16] suggesting that it would be optimal to use those who self-report as night owls, shorten night shifts, and vary shift changes less. However, given the previously mentioned poor judgment of self-rated resilience to sleep loss, employers might benefit from objective tests of judgment and performance during these targeted work times.

There is evidence that a 34 hour "restart" time following a shift with optimal circadian rhythm, lead to recovery of skills as demonstrated by PVT performance skills. The 34 hour restart, however was not found to be adequate in recovery of performance during a simulated night shift rotation.[17] There is as of yet no replacement for adequate sleep time or a proper circadian alignment. However, in the short term and for the purposes of maintaining alertness and performance in personnel required to work after inadequate total sleep time or under conditions of circadian misalignment, pharmacologic options provide some promise.

Bonnet designed a well-controlled study evaluating naps of varying length (0, 2, 4, or 8 hours) and caffeine (400 mg qd or 150 or 300 mg every 6 hours) on performance mood and alertness in complete sleep deprivation.[18] Performance, mood rating, and alertness rating were directly related to the length of prophylactic nap. They found that beyond 24 hours, caffeine lost benefit to performance. They summarized that 2 to 3 hours of nap was equivalent to 150 to 300 mg of caffeine. The 8-hour nap provided increased alertness and performance compared with all other groups.[18] Power napping in lieu of rest breaks alone (no sleep is obtained, only restful wake activity) is essential when workers are lacking sleep. Well-slept individuals should not require napping; rest breaks alone should be adequate in cases of worker fatigue related to emotional, cognitive, or physical stress. The common miss-attribution that one falls asleep during a meeting because of boredom is well known. Workers fall asleep during meetings because of lack of sleep, disrupted sleep, lack of stimulation, and sitting, rather than being in an orthostatic position, which would prevent sleep. However, breaks can allow workers to find individual strategies that work well for him or her.

Scheduled breaks have been associated with reduced accident rate in the work place.[19] Furthermore, breaks may need to be longer for some types of sustained attention work to reduce accident rates and error. Exercise has also been found effective in allaying sleepiness in aviators in a sleep-deprived condition, although the effects were short lived.[20] Although there is anecdotal evidence that exercise is beneficial in allaying fatigue in the work place, there is little data on this, whereas there have been multiple studies on the benefits of exercise on fatigue in illnesses such as multiple sclerosis and cancer. Overall, exercise appears to be a very temporary countermeasure for shift work–related fatigue and sleepiness.

The use of work task variation and increased novelty to facilitate psychological and motor vigilance has not been well examined. Introducing novel activities through the necessity of attention and focus may diminish mental or cognitive fatigue. Variation in task may break up fatigue related to tasks requiring sustained attention and focus. This could be accomplished by introducing the need to vary or rotate work tasks at various intervals for tasks that may be repetitive and intellectually numbing. An example of this would be assembly line work in which a worker may shift tasks from tightening the proverbial widget to clearing the damaged widgets from a widget rejection area. Noise also has been found effective in improving vigilance sleep-deprived individuals,[21] although certainly possible negative consequences on concentration and mood should be a consideration. Variable sound levels and music may be adaptable as antifatigue measures in the work place.

Bright light exposure, particularly blue light, has promise for improving nocturnal performance under a sleep-deprived condition[22] and has been well established as a tool to phase-shift individuals. For shift workers, use of bright light (particularly blue light, which suppresses melatonin) may be beneficial in diminishing sleepiness and fatigue. In one study, combination of bright light and caffeine (at doses of 200 mg at 20:00 and 02:00 hours) was more effective than either treatment alone and was able to minimize the circadian drop in performance across tasks.[23] However, bright light alone does not appear to influence performance as beneficially as a brief nap.

Night shift workers appear to have different eating habits during work than do day shift workers; primarily in the form of eating more regular small meals, increased sugar from soft drinks, and reduced fiber.[24] Additionally, because they are eating at unnatural times with regard to circadian rhythm, they experience lowered glucose and lipid tolerance following a change from day to night shift.[25] Lowden and colleagues[24] recommend several guidelines to facilitate healthier nutrition in shift workers including providing healthy dining facilities with a variety of food choices, and a proper meal break similar to the lunch break enjoyed by day shift workers, avoiding large meals, avoiding or restricting energy intake between midnight and 6 AM, and pre-shift and post-shift meals in lieu of more shift-time meals.[24]

Pharmacologic and nonpharmacologic interventions to modify fatigue and sleepiness suggest some overall improvement in alertness and performance with a variety of agents. Caffeine has proved successful as a counter fatigue measure in driving simulations. Many studies have shown the benefits of caffeine in mitigating the effects of sleep deprivation induced by prolonged total work hours.[26,27] In a large population-based study of 3041 randomly sampled drivers, numerous countermeasures were reported to include stop to take a walk (54%), turn on the radio/stereo (52%), open a window (47%), drink coffee (45%), and to ask passengers to engage in conversation (35%).[28]

In a 12-month open label study, armodafinil effectively diminished sleepiness in 98% of night shift workers during shift or while driving home post-shift.[29] Armodafinil was also found to be associated with decreased sleepiness during night shift and drive home as well as to improve memory and attention compared with placebo. It was not associated with increased sleep onset latency when sleep was desired post-shift (a known problem with amphetamines and methamphetamines).[30] Although amphetamine and methamphetamines are worth note, as they are not clinically indicated for SWSD and there are safer alternatives that have been well studied, they will not be reviewed in the body of this article. Although the data on caffeine and armodafinil are promising, it must be emphasized that there is no evidence that they adequately compensate sleep loss pharmacologically past a few hours of shift. Additionally, they carry some risks and should be used only as an adjunct safely and under supervision of a physician. Although caffeine is not controlled, it does have cardiotoxic properties and has abuse potential.

On the opposite side of alerting and wakefulness, is the importance of facilitating the phase transition when the worker needs to sleep. Nonprescription options that are specific to phase shifting include melatonin and the prescription ramelteon, which have both been found effective in facilitating sleep for shift workers. Although again, meltatonin is regulated in many countries and despite its over-the-counter status it is worthy of review with a treating physician before use.

Preventing burnout by avoiding misaligned shift schedules, providing support, providing training, and awareness of risk factors and educating workers about individual differences cannot be emphasized enough. There is no evidence that any counter fatigue measure can completely reverse the effects of long-term sleep deprivation or circadian misalignment. In addition to errors and injuries including post shift motor vehicle accidents, post–night shift, there is growing evidence that shift work carries other long-term health risks.[31] Although a combination of countermeasures tailored to the individual is optimal, awareness that safety measures must be used as workers are in less optimal conditions and thus at greater risk for error and accident should not be underestimated. Although countermeasures are beneficial in facilitating alertness and performance, they are, according to all studies conducted to date, only temporary solutions to improving worker conditions in the absence of actual sleep time and circadian alignment. Stressful work shift schedules may be because of total work hours, rotating shifts, circadian misalignment, and overall stressful responsibilities because of the potential risks of error from sleepiness and fatigue. Those who feel well supported by their managers and colleagues, more enthusiastic about their job tasks, and less fatigued will have an overall lower rate of burnout than those lacking in these qualities. Some work places offer additional resources, which may allay fatigue such as yoga classes and fitness centers, places for napping, nutritious food options, and strategic lighting. Several large corporations have developed strategies to facilitate naps as a workplace option through nap or quiet rooms.

Respecting sleep and incorporating such programs into the corporate milieu could greatly change the productivity, safety, and health conditions of shift work. Corporations willing to make such moves are also likely to improve social perception of the importance of sleep and healthy behaviors, to be more attractive to potential employees and to influence how sleep is perceived in their communities.

The willingness of several innovative and successful companies to incorporate policies including healthier work schedules and at work options for napping, breaks, healthy dietary option, and better lighting, is promising.

REFERENCES

1. Rosekind MR, Smith RM, Miller DL, et al. Alertness management: strategic naps in operational settings. J Sleep Res 1995;4:62–6.
2. Hursh SR, Van Dongen HP. Fatigue and performance modeling. In: Kryger MH, Roth T, Dement WC, editors. Principals and practices of sleep medicine. 5th edition. St Louis (MO): Elsevier; 2011. p. 745–59.
3. Belenky G, Akerstedt T. Occupational sleep medicine. In: Kryger M, Roth T, Dement WC, editors. Principals and practice of sleep medicine. St Louis (MO): Elsevier Saunders; 2011. p. 734–7.
4. Van Dongen HP, Belenky G. Individual differences in vulnerability to sleep loss in the work environment. Ind Health 2009;47:518–26.
5. Ohayon MM, Dauvilliers Y, Reynolds CF III. Operational definitions and algorithms for excessive sleepiness in the general population: implications for DSM-5 nosology. Arch Gen Psychiatry 2012;69:71–9.
6. Martin JS, Hebert M, Ledoux E, et al. Relationship of chronotype to sleep, light exposure, and work-related fatigue in student workers. Chronobiol Int 2012;29:295–304.
7. Jones CB, Dorrian J, Jay SM, et al. Self-awareness of impairment and the decision to drive after an extended period of wakefulness. Chronobiol Int 2006;23:1253–63.
8. Qureshi AU, Ali AS, Hafeez A, et al. The effect of consecutive extended duty hours on the cognitive and behavioural performance of paediatric medicine residents. J Pak Med Assoc 2010;60:644–9.
9. Ohayon MM, Smolensky MH, Roth T. Consequences of shiftworking on sleep duration, sleepiness, and sleep attacks. Chronobiol Int 2010;27:575–89.
10. Ellen RL, Marshall SC, Palayew M, et al. Systematic review of motor vehicle crash risk in persons with sleep apnea. J Clin Sleep Med 2006;2:193–200.
11. Aldrich MS. Automobile accidents in patients with sleep disorders. Sleep 1989;12:487–94.
12. Hublin C, Partinen M, Koskenvuo M, et al. Sleep and mortality: a population-based 22-year follow-up study. Sleep 2007;30:1245–53.
13. Ferrie JE, Shipley MJ, Cappuccio FP, et al. A prospective study of change in sleep duration: associations with mortality in the Whitehall II cohort. Sleep 2007;30:1659–66.
14. Pack AI, Pack AM, Rodgman E, et al. Characteristics of crashes attributed to the driver having fallen asleep. Accid Anal Prev 1995;27:769–75.
15. Mitler MM, Carskadon MA, Czeisler CA, et al. Catastrophes, sleep, and public policy: consensus report. Sleep 1988;11:100–9.
16. Akerstedt T. Work hours and sleepiness. Neurophysiol Clin 1995;25:367–75.
17. Van Dongen HP, Belenky G, Vila BJ. The efficacy of a restart break for recycling with optimal performance depends critically on circadian timing. Sleep 2011;34:917–29.
18. Bonnet MH, Gomez S, Wirth O, et al. The use of caffeine versus prophylactic naps in sustained performance. Sleep 1995;18:97–104.
19. Arlinghaus A, Lombardi DA, Courtney TK, et al. The effect of rest breaks on time to injury - a study on work-related ladder-fall injuries in the United States. Scand J Work Environ Health 2012;38:560–7.
20. LeDuc PA Jr, Caldwell JA Jr, Ruyak PS. The effects of exercise as a countermeasure for fatigue in sleep-deprived aviators. Mil Psychol 2000;12:249–66.
21. Wilkinson RT. Interaction of noise with knowledge of results and sleep deprivation. J Exp Psychol 1963;66:332–7.
22. Yokoi M, Aoki K, Shimomura Y, et al. Exposure to bright light modifies HRV responses to mental tasks during nocturnal sleep deprivation. J Physiol Anthropol 2006;25:153–61.
23. Wright KP, Badia P, Myers BL, et al. Combination of bright light and caffeine as a countermeasure for impaired alertness and performance during extended sleep deprivation. J Sleep Res 1997;6:26–35.
24. Lowden A, Moreno C, Holmback U, et al. Eating and shift work - effects on habits, metabolism and performance. Scand J Work Environ Health 2010;36:150–62.
25. Hampton SM, Morgan LM, Lawrence N, et al. Postprandial hormone and metabolic responses in simulated shift work. J Endocrinol 1996;151:259–67.
26. Benitez PL, Kamimori GH, Balkin TJ, et al. Modeling fatigue over sleep deprivation, circadian rhythm, and caffeine with a minimal performance inhibitor model. Meth Enzymol 2009;454:405–21.
27. Beaumont M, Batejat D, Pierard C, et al. Slow release caffeine and prolonged (64-h) continuous wakefulness: effects on vigilance and cognitive performance. J Sleep Res 2001;10:265–76.
28. Anund A, Kecklund G, Peters B, et al. Driver sleepiness and individual differences in preferences for countermeasures. J Sleep Res 2008;17:16–22.

29. Schwartz JR, Khan A, McCall WV, et al. Tolerability and efficacy of armodafinil in naive patients with excessive sleepiness associated with obstructive sleep apnea, shift work disorder, or narcolepsy: a 12-month, open-label, flexible-dose study with an extension period. J Clin Sleep Med 2010;6:450–7.

30. Czeisler CA, Walsh JK, Wesnes KA, et al. Armodafinil for treatment of excessive sleepiness associated with shift work disorder: a randomized controlled study. Mayo Clin Proc 2009;84:958–72.

31. Costa G. The impact of shift and night work on health. Appl Ergon 1996;27:9–16.

Medical Management of Fatigue

Amir Sharafkhaneh, MD, PhD[a,b,*],
Suryakanta Velamuri, MD[a,b], Jose Melendez, MD[a,b],
Farah Akhtar, MD[a,b], Max Hirshkowitz, PhD[a,b,c]

KEYWORDS

- Congestive heart failure • Chronic obstructive pulmonary disease • Asthma • Chronic renal failure
- Chronic liver failure • Anemia

KEY POINTS

- Fatigue is frequently reported in chronic medical conditions including cardiovascular, respiratory, renal, and hepatic diseases.
- Improvement of the primary condition positively affects health-related quality of life and fatigue.
- Interventions to achieve exercise rehabilitation robustly affect the fatigue in these patients.
- Improving sleep may improve the quality of life and fatigue.

INTRODUCTION

Fatigue is a near-universal presentation in patients with chronic medical conditions. Variety of pathophysiologic mechanisms is proposed as the link between the chronic conditions and fatigue. Interventions that improve the underlying pathophysiology of these chronic medical conditions result in improvement of quality of life and fatigue. In addition, interventions like rehabilitation that directly work on skeletal muscles, emotional well-being, nutrition, and sleep may improve fatigue. Chronic medical conditions are frequently associated with insomnia and sleep disordered breathing. Interventions that improve sleep in these patients may positively affect the quality of life and fatigue. This article discusses organ-specific interventions that may affect fatigue. The pharmacologic therapies that may improve fatigue are also discussed.

DISEASE-SPECIFIC MANAGEMENT

Medical Management of Cardiac Diseases and Their Effects on Fatigue

Heart failure remains the most common cause of hospitalization and morbidity/mortality in the elderly population.[1] Its associated symptoms of dyspnea, lower extremity edema, and fatigue often prove debilitating to those affected. Although these symptoms may cause functional limitations, they also significantly affect patients' psychological and social welfare.

Current recommended pharmacotherapy for heart failure includes angiotensin-converting enzyme inhibitor (ACE-I), angiotensin receptor blocker (ARB), β-blocker, aldosterone antagonist, oral nitrates, and hydralazine (in African-American patients), diuretics, digoxin, and rehabilitation.[2] Randomized trials of lisinopril, an ACE-I, in patients with heart failure showed improvement in

[a] Section of Pulmonary and Critical Care and Sleep Medicine, Baylor College of Medicine, Houston, TX, USA; [b] Sleep Disorders & Research Center, Michael E.DeBakey VA Medical Center, Baylor College of Medicine, Houston, TX, USA; [c] Menninger Department of Psychiatry, Baylor College of Medicine, Houston, TX, USA
* Corresponding author. Baylor College of Medicine, MEDVA Medical Center Building, 100 (111i), Houston, TX 77030.
E-mail address: amirs@bcm.edu

Sleep Med Clin 8 (2013) 265–276
http://dx.doi.org/10.1016/j.jsmc.2013.04.002
1556-407X/13/$ – see front matter Published by Elsevier Inc.

exercise and fatigue.[3–5] Addition of valsartan (an ARB) to regular heart failure therapy improved fatigue.[6] In contrast, a large, randomized, placebo-controlled trail of ibesartan did not show significant improvement in disease-specific quality of life and fatigue.[7]

β-Blockers are the mainstay of therapy in congestive heart failure (CHF).[2] There have been multiple studies evaluating fatigue secondary to β-blocker use. Although fatigue was a frequent cause for β-blocker cessation in some, others failed to find a significant correlation between its use and fatigue. In a large study of carvedilol in daily practice, fatigue was reported in 5% to 6.5% of patients.[8] In contrast, in Beta-Blocker Evaluation of Survival Trial (BEST) trial, the prevalence of fatigue between the active arm receiving bucindolol and placebo was similar.[9] A quantitative review of randomized trials tested β-blockers in myocardial infarctions, heart failure, and hypertension to determine the association of β-blockers with depressive symptoms, fatigue, and sexual dysfunction.[10] The 15 trials analyzed involved more than 35,000 subjects. β-Blocker use was associated with a small significant annual increase in risk of reported fatigue equivalent to 1 additional report of fatigue for every 57 patients treated per year with β-blockers. The risk associated with reported fatigue was significantly higher for early-generation than for late-generation β-blockers ($P = .04$). As with any medication, the risk of any adverse effects must be weighed against the benefits it provides.

A variety of other pharmacologic interventions has been tested in patients with heart failure. Levosimendan is a calcium sensitizer that enhances myocardial contractility without increasing myocardial oxygen use. It improves cardiac contractility and has been used in patients with severe systolic heart failure. In a randomized trial of intermittent levosimendan, various outcomes including dyspnea and fatigue and ejection fraction improved significantly.[11] In a randomized, double-blinded, placebo-controlled study, Kumar and colleagues[12] evaluated the effects of a combination of ubiquinol and carnitine in various outcomes in patients with systolic heart failure. Patients in the active arm of the study had significant improvement in fatigue, dyspnea, palpitation, and 6-minute walk test.[12] In a trial of *Crataegus* extract (WS 1442) in 588 patients with New York Heart Association class II who received the agent compared with a comparative group of 364 patients for 2 years, the active group showed significant improvement in fatigue, dyspnea, and palpitations.[13] The groups in the study were not comparable in regard to baseline medications. In a randomized trial of vasopressin antagonism in 4133 patients admitted to hospital with acute heart failure, tolvaptan reduced physician-assessed fatigue during the hospital stay.[14]

Cardiac fatigue may be partially caused by abnormal muscle histology, metabolism, and quantity in addition to endothelial dysfunction, and this has formed the foundation for interventions such as muscle exercise training and respiratory muscle training. These actions can potentially improve all the noted muscular abnormalities in addition to endothelial function of the peripheral circulation.[15] Through these improvements, the sensation of fatigue is therefore reduced as well. Exercise training has also been shown to reduce the level of ventilation during exercise, to reduce the degree of sympathoexcitation, and to correct partial abnormalities in heart rate variability. Improvement in muscle strength and reduction of muscle fatigability in part may explain the improvement in fatigue with exercise rehabilitation in patients with heart failure.[16] An extensive review of trials of cardiac rehabilitation showed decreased hospitalization and improved quality of life.[17] Various regimens include treadmill or bicycle exercise, interval exercise, training of individual extremities, or specific muscle strength training. In a randomized, controlled, double-blind study of inspiratory muscle training in patients with heart failure, quality of life, peripheral muscle strength, and fatigue significantly improved with intervention.[18] In a randomized trial of home-based exercise training, Wall and colleagues[19] reported improvement in fatigue and dyspnea with home-based exercise intervention. In a randomized study of exercise rehabilitation for chronic obstructive pulmonary disease (COPD) in patients with CHF and COPD, Evans and colleagues[20] reported comparable improvement in fatigue in both group of study subjects. Pozehl and colleagues[21] similarly reported significant improvement in fatigue using the Piper Fatigue Scale in a randomized trial of aerobic and resistance training 3 times weekly in patients with systolic heart failure. In contrast with the exercise rehabilitation, a 12-week randomized trial of tai chi improved depressive symptoms but not fatigue.[22] However, physical fatigue changes correlated with depressive symptoms changes.[22] In summary, various programs of exercise rehabilitation improve fatigue in patients with heart failure.

Education of patients with chronic medical conditions plays an important role in long-term management of these patients. In an education intervention study, Albert and colleagues[23] compared standard education (SE) during discharge from a CHF admission with standard education and video education (SE + VE) on various clinical outcomes. In the follow-up phone evaluation, the individuals randomized to SE + VE had significantly less profound fatigue with exertion compared with the SE group.

Nutritional restrictions in salt and water intake are recommended by American College of Cardiology and American Heart Association and European Society of Cardiology.[24,25] Colin and colleagues in a randomized trial evaluated effect of salt and water–restricted diet on symptoms, leg edema, and fatigue. The salt-restricted group showed significant reduction in fatigue and edema in 6 months.[26]

Sleep disorders are prevalent in patients with heart failure.[27] Sleep disordered breathing is common in these patients.[28] In a randomized, double-blind, cross-over trial in patients with heart failure and central sleep apnea (CSA), 6 nights of a nightly single dose of acetazolamide 1 hour before bedtime improved CSA, overall quality of life, and fatigue.[28] Javaheri[29] reported improvement with theophylline in patients with heart failure and CSA, but data related to quality of life and fatigue were not provided. Overnight administration of O_2 similarly improved hypoxia but did not affect the daytime symptoms.[30] Thus, further information on effect of treatment of CSA in heart failure–related fatigue is required.

Medical Management of Respiratory Diseases and Their Effects on Fatigue

COPD

Medical management of COPD is intended to improve expiratory flow and thereby improve exercise capacity and quality of life. Correlation between expiratory flow impairment and indices of quality of life, fatigue, and depressive symptoms is imperfect. Thus, improvement in expiratory flow limitation with bronchodilators may not correlate linearly with improvements in quality of life, fatigue, and depressive symptoms. Optimal bronchodilation by long-acting bronchodilators is the first step in the treatment of patients with COPD. However; greater treatment effects (eg, improvements in exercise performance, symptoms, and health-related quality of life including fatigue) are often achieved with the addition of pulmonary rehabilitation.[31] Comprehensive pulmonary rehabilitation programs are designed to tackle the systemic consequences of COPD, as well as the behavioral and educational deficiencies observed in many patients.[32]

Long-acting inhalational anticholinergics like tiotropium and aclidinium are major therapeutic options in the management of stable COPD.

Randomized trials of these agents showed improvement in lung function, exercise capacity, quality of life, dyspnea, COPD exacerbation, and nocturnal oxygen desaturations.[33–42] Evaluation of fatigue using fatigue-specific instruments was not part of the trials and thus data are not available. However, improvement in quality of life, exercise capacity, and dyspnea may indirectly imply some degree of improvement in fatigue.

Long-acting beta agonists like salmeterol, formoterol, and indacaterol are approved agents for management of stable COPD. Randomized trials show improvement in various objective and patient-reported outcomes including exercise capacity and quality of life. The effect of the medications on fatigue is not well studied. In a randomized clinical trial of indacaterol, add-on therapy compared with placebo, 6-minute walk test, quality of life, and fatigue improved.[43]

Inhaled corticosteroids alone or in combination are widely used for management of stable COPD. The Inhaled Steroids in Obstructive Lung Disease in Europe (ISOLDE) trial showed faster decline in quality of life (including the SF-36 with energy/ vitality domain) in patients on placebo compared with inhaled steroid.[44] Most improvements seen with inhaled steroids are in the form of combination therapy with long-acting beta-2 agonists. The current products available are fluticasone/ salmeterol, budesonide/formoterol, and mometasone/formoterol (only approved for asthma). The combination therapy improves lung function, exercise capacity, and quality of life, and reduces exacerbations.[45–50] Spencer and Anderson[51] reported on improvement in dyspnea and fatigue with the use of combination of fluticasone/salmeterol in patients with stable COPD. In summary, current pharmacotherapeutic options improve many pathophysiologic aspects of COPD and improve quality of life. However, evaluation of their effects on fatigue has been limited.

Since the first controlled trials on pulmonary rehabilitation in the mid-1970s (for review see Casaburi and Petty[32]) and in the early 1980s, pulmonary rehabilitation has been proved to result in clinically significant improvements in more than 20 methodologically well-designed randomized controlled trials.[52] According to the World Health Organization's Global Initiative for Chronic Obstructive Lung Disease (GOLD) consensus document on the management of COPD, pulmonary rehabilitation should be considered in patients with an forced expiratory volume in 1 second (FEV_1) less than 80% of the predicted value. In addition, most national and international guidelines consider pulmonary rehabilitation an important treatment option.[52–54] Various studies show improvement in fatigue with exercise rehabilitation program in patients with COPD.[20,53,55]

Interstitial lung diseases

Pulmonary rehabilitation is effective in improving exercise and quality of life in patients with COPD, but the data on efficacy of pulmonary rehabilitation in restrictive lung disease are limited. In a small group of patients with pulmonary fibrosis, pulmonary rehabilitation improved exercise endurance and quality of life, and reduce hospital admissions.[56,57] However, the effect of pulmonary rehabilitation on fatigue in patients with interstitial lung diseases is not well studied.

Medical Management of Renal Diseases and Their Effects on Fatigue

Fatigue is a common complaint among patients with chronic kidney disorders (CKDs) and among patients on dialysis. It is often the most debilitating symptom that contributes to a poor quality of life in these patients.[58,59]

To know how to manage fatigue among patients with renal disorders, it is important to consider the possible causes of this symptom in patients with renal disease. Although no single cause of fatigue in these patients is apparent, it is likely that several factors contribute to development of fatigue. A large contributor to fatigue in patients with CKD is the presence of anemia. Anemia is seen in a significant number (up to 14.7%) of patients with chronic kidney disease not on dialysis.[60] Anemia in these patients is caused by decreased production of erythropoietin. In addition to the presence of anemia, there seems to be impairment in oxygen delivery and oxygen extraction in patients with CKD.[61] In a healthy person with induced anemia, there is usually an increase in cardiac output, which helps maintain a steady oxygen delivery despite the anemia. However, in patients with CKD, there is an insufficient increase in cardiac output. Oxygen extraction at the tissue level also does not increase to compensate for the decrease in oxygen delivery. Decreased oxygen delivery caused by anemia and inadequate compensatory increase in cardiac output combined with a lack of compensatory increase in oxygen extraction results in decreased tissue oxygenation and can lead to fatigue.

Another important consideration in evaluating fatigue in patients with renal disease is the contribution of psychological conditions. Depression is common among patients with CKD and among patients on dialysis.[62,63] The presence of depression in patients with CKD is higher than in patients with other chronic illnesses like congestive heart failure.[64] In a large observational study of dialysis patients in the United States, Boulware and colleagues[65] reported a prevalence of depressive symptoms ranging from 19% to 24%, which is similar to other comparative studies. In a study of 47 patients in India undergoing hemodialysis, depression assessed by the Beck Depression Inventory Questionnaire was present in as many as 72.3% of patients, with 12.6% having severe depression. A positive correlation was found between presence of fatigue and depression in this study.[63]

The third factor that likely plays a role in the development of fatigue among patients with CKD is the presence of concomitant sleep disorders.[63] Daytime sleepiness has been reported in 11.8% to 31% of patients on hemodialysis.[66–68] Restless legs syndrome (RLS) is common among patients with CKD.

Management of fatigue in patients with CKD should focus on the pathophysiologic mechanisms of fatigue in these patients. Treatments designed to improve tissue oxygenation, treatment of depression and other psychological disorders, and treatment of underlying sleep disorders are key in the management of fatigue.

The role of erythropoiesis-stimulating agents in the treatment of anemia in patients with CKD and on dialysis has been extensively studied. However, most trials in patients with CKD not on dialysis were non–placebo controlled or open labeled. A large multicenter trial (The Trial to Reduce cardiovascular Events with Aranesp [darbepoetin alfa] Therapy [TREAT] trial) of 4038 patients in 24 countries studied the effect of darbepoetin alfa in patients with diabetes and chronic kidney disease with anemia. The targeted hemoglobin level in this trial was 13 g/dL. There was no difference seen in the primary end point of cardiovascular morbidity and mortality and an increased risk of stroke in patients treated with darbepoetin. A detailed analysis of health-related quality-of-life measures for fatigue, energy, and physical function was done. Results showed that fatigue was significantly improved in patients who received darbepoetin with no difference in energy or physical function scores initially. This improvement remained sustained over the 2-year follow-up period. Given increased risk of stroke and no difference in cardiovascular outcomes, the decision to use erythropoiesis-stimulating agents in patients with CKD and fatigue should be individualized and discussed with the patient.[69]

L-Carnitine has been studied to decrease the effects of fatigue in patients with CKD. L-Carnitine is important for muscle function and has been found to be deficient in patients on hemodialysis

(HD). L-Carnitine supplementation has been found to be helpful in relieving fatigue in patients who are resistant to epoetin therapy in some studies, but the overall data show inconclusive results.[70]

Physical exercise has been shown to decrease fatigue in other medical disorders. Chang and colleagues[71] showed that, in a study of 40 patients, lower extremity resistance exercise training for 12 weeks during hemodialysis using ankle weights improved self-reported physical functioning as well as a trend toward a reduction in fatigue in the groups that were assigned to exercise.[72] Anabolic steroids and resistance exercise similarly produced anabolic effects in patients with chronic renal disease.[21] Yoga and acupressure are also beneficial in reducing fatigue in patients with HD. In a small randomized trial of 39 patients on hemodialysis, 30 minutes of yoga twice a week for 3 months showed a 55% improvement in fatigue compared with the placebo group.

Treatment of depression in patients with CKD is essential. All patients undergoing hemodialysis should be screened for depression with a screening scale like the Beck Depression Inventory (BDI). For those patients who meet the criteria for depression, therapy should be initiated. Nonpharmacologic therapies should be considered in patients with CKD and depression/fatigue. Studies have shown that increased frequency of hemodialysis (up to 6 times a week) decreased the BDI score as well as improving quality-of-life/fatigue scores.[73,74] Cognitive behavior therapy (CBT) is another nonpharmacologic option to treat depression in patients with CKD. In a study of 85 patients, Duarte and colleagues[75] found that CBT reduced depression scores and improved SF-36 quality-of-life and fatigue scores. Pharmacologic therapy for depression includes treatment with selective serotonin reuptake inhibitors or tricyclic antidepressants. Given the higher incidence of cardiovascular morbidity and mortality in patients with renal disorders, physicians need to be aware of the cardiac side effects of antidepressants. However, few good studies have looked at the pharmacotherapy for depression among patients with CKD or dialysis. Small uncontrolled studies and 1 small (n = 14) randomized study of antidepressants in patients on dialysis showed improvement in depression scores but unclear long-term outcomes. A large randomized controlled trial is underway to examine the effect of antidepressants on depression, fatigue, and quality of life in patients with CKD.[64]

Treatment of sleep disorders like insomnia, obstructive sleep apnea, and RLS can help improve fatigue and overall well-being in patients with CKD. However, there is a paucity of good studies assessing the effect of treatment of sleep disorders in patients with CKD and HD on the symptoms of fatigue or other outcomes.

Fatigue is common in patients with chronic kidney diseases and has multifactorial causes. Therefore, assessment for and treatment of fatigue should also be multifactorial .[76]

Liver Diseases

Effects on fatigue

As in renal disorders, fatigue is a predominant and presenting symptom in many liver disorders.[77] It is most prominent in cholestatic liver diseases, especially primary biliary cirrhosis (PBC). Fatigue can occur in 65% to 85% of patients with cholestatic liver diseases.[78] It is seen to occur almost as commonly in other cholestatic disorders like primary sclerosing cholangitis and drug-induced cholangitis. In these cholestatic disorders, it is not only the most common symptom, it is also the most disabling symptom.[79] Patients report their health-related quality of life to be adversely affected by this debilitating fatigue.

In PBC, the degree of fatigue does not correlate with autoantibody levels, histologic stage of disease, or with degree of liver damage. Fatigue in PBC strongly correlates with poor sleep hygiene and with excessive daytime sleepiness in the absence of sleep disordered breathing.[80] In another study of 42 early-stage patients with PBC, 29% had RLS and 50% of patients tested with leg actigraphy had periodic leg movement disorder as well.[81] In addition, the degree of fatigue in patients with PBC is related to autonomic dysfunction, which may also correlate with the increased mortality seen in patients with PBC and fatigue.[80]

Fatigue is also seen predominantly in other hepatic disorders like autoimmune hepatitis and parallels the activity of the disease. In viral hepatitis, fatigue is a common symptom during acute hepatitis phases. However, the data regarding prevalence of fatigue in chronic viral hepatitis are mixed. In chronic hepatitis C infection, patients' reporting of fatigue is related to their awareness of the diagnosis.[82] In chronic hepatitis B infection, there is no increased prevalence of fatigue as a presenting symptom.

In nonalcoholic fatty liver disease (NAFLD), one of the most common liver disorders in the Western world, systemic symptoms are frequently the presenting symptoms rather than symptoms directly of their liver disease. Of these symptoms, fatigue and excessive daytime sleepiness are the most common. In a cohort of patients with chronic liver diseases in Newcastle, United Kingdom, 44% of patients with NAFLD had Fatigue Impact Scale

Scores greater than 40, indicating severe fatigue. Fatigue in NAFLD is not related to the severity of disease. It correlates more with symptoms of daytime sleepiness and autonomic dysfunction.[83]

In patients with end-stage liver disease and cirrhosis undergoing transplant evaluation, increased fatigue levels are seen. Fatigue in these patients is related to the severity of cirrhosis, presence of ascites, and to the presence of hepatic encephalopathy. In these patients, fatigue in part seems to be related to increased incidence of anxiety and depression as well. Low cortisol, anemia, and impaired renal function were also independent predictors of fatigue.[84]

Managing the fatigue

In the management of fatigue in liver diseases, specific therapies targeting fatigue have not been studied. Therefore, general measures are important in managing this symptom. An important first step is for the treating physician to screen for the presence of this symptom in patients with chronic liver diseases. For most patients, this is the most debilitating symptom and acknowledging and validating their symptoms is important. Patients should be assessed for any concomitant disorders that may be contributing to their symptoms of fatigue, especially hypothyroidism.

Excessive daytime sleepiness correlates directly with the level of fatigue in patients with liver diseases. Poor sleep hygiene with prolonged sleep latency and early morning awakenings are seen frequently in patients with PBC.[85] This finding correlated with levels and timing of pruritus. Treatments targeting pruritus and addressing sleep hygiene in these patients can improve sleep quality and improve fatigue.

Patients with fatigue and excessive daytime sleepiness should be screened for sleep-related breathing disorders (SBD). In patients with associated SBD, treatment with positive-pressure therapy is recommended. In patients without SBD, treatment with alerting agents such as modafinil may be an option. In a study by Gan and colleagues, 42 patients with PBC and severe fatigue with excessive daytime sleepiness were treated with 100 to 200 mg of modafinil. Thirty-one (74%) of these patients showed immediate improvement in their fatigue within 3 days and were continued on therapy. In long-term follow-up for up to 18 months, 25 patients continued with therapy with minimal side effects and sustained improvement in fatigue and daytime activity levels.

Assessment for and treatment of concomitant RLS in patients with PBC can help improve fatigue as well. In a study in which 11 patients with symptomatic RLS, fatigue, and PBC were treated with dopamine agonist therapies, 63% of patients who took the therapy noted a clear benefit in their symptoms of RLS and improvement in fatigue as well.[81]

The effect of antiviral therapy for chronic hepatitis C on fatigue was analyzed as a part of the Virahep-C study. Fatigue measurements were taken before, during, and after therapy. The number of patients reporting fatigue as well as the severity of fatigue worsened while patients were on treatment with interferon and ribavirin. Fatigue severity remained high for the duration of therapy. After completion of therapy, the prevalence of fatigue decreased and, by 12 weeks, was lower than at baseline, especially in those who achieved a sustained viral response.[86]

The effect of liver transplantation on fatigue in patients with cirrhosis has also been studied. In 60 patients who underwent liver transplantation, overall Fatigue Impact Scale score improved 1 year after transplantation compared with pretransplant levels. However, up to 50% of patients had persistent physical fatigue compared with controls. Those patients who had persistent fatigue after transplantation had higher physical, psychosocial, and total Fatigue Impact Scale Scores at baseline (pretransplant) and had more frequent or significant depression.[84]

Fatigue in liver diseases is common. However, distinct pathogenetic causes have not been defined. Therefore, management of fatigue in these patients has to be multidimensional. Further studies with specific targeted therapies to improve fatigue in patients with chronic liver diseases will be useful.

NON–DISEASE-SPECIFIC PHARMACOTHERAPY FOR FATIGUE
Overview

Using substances to augment wakefulness reportedly dates back to 1900 BC when Mesoamerican priests began using chocolate. By the thirteenth century, the Aztecs had attributed the appearance of Theobroma cacao to the god Quetzalcoatl who brought it from paradise. On the other side of the world, the discovery of coffee in the ninth century was attributed to a goat herder named Kaldi who was led to it by his goats dancing in the moonlight.

Using stimulants to offset sleepiness and manage fatigue deserves careful consideration of the risks and benefits. On the risk side of the equation, drug (or substance) side effects are typically considered, and, on the benefit side, improvement in functioning and quality of life are considered. However, some side effects may not yet be fully known. Furthermore, the absence of acute adverse reactions to drugs does not reliably predict long-term side effects. Side effects that produce permanent damage are weighted more heavily for risk than those from which recovery is rapid. Benefits may range from simply economic (eg, working longer shifts to make more money) to being essential for deriving any enjoyment from life overall (eg, severe hypersomnia). The balancing of risks versus benefits becomes more complicated when the task being performed is essential and time critical (eg, searching for earthquake survivors at 4 AM) or extremely difficult (performing a delicate surgery).

Short-term pharmacologic intervention, particularly using central nervous system stimulants, improves alertness and mental acuity, and can prevent inadvertent sleep onset. The key term here is short term. The good-practice, ideal solution involves maintaining adequate sleep and avoiding circadian misalignments. Nonetheless, individuals suffering fatigue provoked by pathologic stressors have fatigue even when adhering to good-practice guidelines. In such cases, the physician must tailor each individual's therapy by considering all of the known (1) risks, (2) benefits, (3) potential interactions with other medications, and (4) contraindications because of comorbid disease. Pharmacotherapy for medical fatigue management is an important part of the overall approach but must be applied with care.

Psychostimulants

Caffeine and theobromine (the methylxanthines)

Caffeine and theobromine assert their stimulant actions by antagonizing brain adenosine receptors.[87] A typical dose from brewed coffee is 100 to 150 mg. A 50-g dark chocolate candy bar has 30 to 40 mg. Caffeine has a half-life of 3 to 7 hours. It improves attention, reaction time, and cognitive performance in sleep-deprived/sleep-restricted normal volunteers. Caffeine and/or theobromine are readily available in beverages (coffee, tea, cola, hot cocoa, and caffeinated water), over-the-counter pills (immediate or time released), gum, candy, and skin creams. Side effects include insomnia, nervousness and restlessness, nausea, anxiety, agitation, tinnitus, and vomiting. Caffeine increases heart rate and respiration. In some individuals it can provoke chest pain and irregular heartbeat.[88] Lethal dose is estimated at approximately 3 g.

Alerting over-the-counter medicines and food additives

Many over-the-counter medicines contain caffeine. However, other substances, such as taurine (in energy drinks), ephedrine, ephedra, and pseudoephedrine (in cold medicines and protein drinks) also produce an alerting response but overall safety is not fully known.

Prescription stimulants

Catacholaminergic stimulants represent the traditional psychostimulants used to promote wakefulness. These drugs predominantly affect catecholamines (dopamine and norepinephrine) by provoking synaptic release and reuptake blockade. Medications acting through these mechanisms include amphetamines and their congeners (eg, methylphenidate). Dopamine and norepinephrine affect cognition, reward, motivation, activity level, attention, and memory. They also profoundly increase wakefulness. Because dopamine plays a major role in reward-seeking behavior, it can induce automatic, obsessive, stereotypic, and compulsive drug-seeking behaviors.

Amphetamines and amphetaminelike stimulants (amphetamine, amphetamine salts, dextroamphetamine, methamphetamine, and methylphenidate) increase catacholaminergic neurotransmitter levels by rupturing presynaptic vesicles and subsequently blocking presynaptic reuptake. They acutely increase levels of dopamine, norepinephrine and serotonin but continued high-dose use can produce depletion.[89,90] The various medications differ with respect to half-life, central versus peripheral action, neurotransmitter specificity, and abuse potential. For example, methylphenidate has a shorter half-life (2–4 hours) compared with amphetamines (8–16 hours) and a lower abuse potential.[91,92] Side effects include headaches, irritability, nervousness, insomnia, anorexia, nausea, vomiting, sweating, and tremors. Some people experience irregular heartbeat and palpitations. In rare cases, these drugs can provoke psychosis and orofacial dyskinesia.[93] Long-term abuse can produce Parkinson disease–like symptoms and dementia.

Noradrenergic reuptake inhibitors can also improve alertness (eg, atomoxetine, reboxetine, viloxazine). Side effects include tachycardia and hypertension, especially at high doses.[94,95] Modafinil (and its right-handed or R enantiomer, armodafinil) is an alternative stimulant. The mechanism is not completely understood. Like other stimulant medications, these compounds enhance catecholamine release and activate norepinephrine and dopamine systems.[96–98] However, unlike the traditional psychostimulants, modafinil and armodafinil seem to inhibit gamma-aminobutyric acid (GABA) transmission and increase hypothalamic histamine levels.[99,100] Modafinil's common side effects include nausea, diarrhea, nervousness, insomnia, and headache. In addition, tachycardia and hypertension occur in some patients, and rare cases are reported in which a life-threatening rash developed.

Soporifics and Chronobiotics

In some cases, fatigue management can benefit from aggressively treating insomnia. A vicious cycle can develop in which poor sleep exacerbates an illness and the illness adversely affects sleep. There are a wide variety of benzodiazepines (BZDs) and BZD receptor agonists (BZRAs) approved for treating insomnia. BZDs approved for insomnia include triazolam, temazepam, estazolam, quazepam, and flurazepam. BZRAs include eszopiclone, zaleplon, and zolpidem. These drugs work primarily through the GABA and BZD mechanisms but differ with respect to half-life.[101] Side effects include headache, morning carryover sedation, amnesia, confusion, and sleepwalking (complex behaviors during sleep).

Another therapeutic avenue for treating insomnia capitalizes on the soporific effects of central histamine blockade. One medication approved for insomnia treatment is a low-dose formulation of doxepin. However, many drugs with antihistaminergic properties are commonly used off-label to promote sleep, including diphenhydramine, trazodone, mirtazepine, amitriptyline, doxepin, quitiapine, and gabapentine. Side effects vary and use of nonapproved medications is discouraged.[102]

Herbal preparations that may or may not have sleep promoting effects include ashwagandha, chamomile, lavender, gotukola, hawthorn, hops, kava, mullein, passionflower, sage, lemon balm, catnip, skullcap, pulsatilla, St John wort, and hops.[103] These herbs, often brewed as tea (but sometimes eaten), reputedly have mildly sedative properties. However, randomized trials and complete side effect profiles are lacking in most cases. In the past, unregulated food additives like L-tryptophan were later found to be associated with serious adverse events. Until more scientific data are available, using these preparations is not advised.

With improved understanding of the role of circadian rhythms in regulating sleep and wakefulness, individuals and clinicians have looked to melatonin and melatonin agonists as a vehicle for improving sleep. For many years there seemed to be problems with melatonin source, purity, and concentration because it was classed as a food additive and therefore not subject to stringent regulation. These difficulties seem to have been resolved. There is also now available pharmaceutical-grade melatonin (Circadin) and a prescription melatonin agonist (ramelteon).[102]

SUMMARY

Fatigue is frequently reported in chronic medical conditions including cardiovascular, respiratory, renal, and hepatic diseases. Improvement of the primary condition positively affects health-related quality of life and fatigue. Interventions to achieve exercise rehabilitation robustly affect the fatigue in these patients. In addition, improving sleep may improve the quality of life and fatigue.

In some cases, medical management may use wake-promoting medications. The risks and benefits must be carefully weighed. When insomnia is contributing significantly to the overall fatigue, pharmacotherapy may be appropriate. It is prudent to adhere to product indications. However, the clinical picture is often complicated by potential interactions with other medications and contraindications because of the comorbid disease producing the fatigue. Many individuals experiencing fatigue use over-the-counter medicines and caffeine. It is important for the physician to be aware of any self-medication when attempting fatigue management.

REFERENCES

1. Fini A, de Almeida Lopes Monteiro da Cruz D. Characteristics of fatigue in heart failure patients: a literature review. Rev Lat Am Enfermagem 2009;17:557–65.
2. Lindenfeld J, Albert NM, Boehmer JP, et al. HFSA 2010 comprehensive heart failure practice guideline. J Card Fail 2010;16:e1–194.
3. Beller B, Bulle T, Bourge RC, et al. Lisinopril versus placebo in the treatment of heart failure: the Lisinopril Heart Failure Study Group. J Clin Pharmacol 1995;35:673–80.
4. Giles TD, Katz R, Sullivan JM, et al. Short- and long-acting angiotensin-converting enzyme inhibitors: a randomized trial of lisinopril versus captopril in the treatment of congestive heart failure. The Multicenter Lisinopril-Captopril Congestive Heart Failure Study Group. J Am Coll Cardiol 1989;13:1240–7.
5. Lewis GR. Comparison of lisinopril versus placebo for congestive heart failure. Am J Cardiol 1989;63:12D–6D.
6. Cohn JN, Tognoni G. A randomized trial of the angiotensin-receptor blocker valsartan in chronic heart failure. N Engl J Med 2001;345:1667–75.
7. Rector TS, Carson PE, Anand IS, et al. Assessment of long-term effects of irbesartan on heart failure with preserved ejection fraction as measured by the Minnesota Living with Heart Failure questionnaire in the Irbesartan in Heart Failure with Preserved Systolic Function (I-PRESERVE) trial. Circ Heart Fail 2012;5:217–25.

8. Lainscak M, Moullet C, Schon N, et al. Treatment of chronic heart failure with carvedilol in daily practice: the SATELLITE survey experience. Int J Cardiol 2007;122:149–55.

9. Beta-Blocker Evaluation of Survival Trial Investigators. A trial of the beta-blocker bucindolol in patients with advanced chronic heart failure. N Engl J Med 2001;344:1659–67.

10. Ko DT, Hebert PR, Coffey CS, Sedrakyan A, Curtis JP, Krumholz HM. Beta-blocker therapy and symptoms of depression, fatigue, and sexual dysfunction. JAMA 2002 Jul 17;288(3):351–7.

11. Mavrogeni S, Giamouzis G, Papadopoulou E, et al. A 6-month follow-up of intermittent levosimendan administration effect on systolic function, specific activity questionnaire, and arrhythmia in advanced heart failure. J Card Fail 2007;13:556–9.

12. Kumar A, Singh RB, Saxena M, et al. Effect of Carni Q-Gel (ubiquinol and carnitine) on cytokines in patients with heart failure in the Tishcon study. Acta Cardiol 2007;62:349–54.

13. Habs M. Prospective, comparative cohort studies and their contribution to the benefit assessments of therapeutic options: heart failure treatment with and without Hawthorn special extract WS 1442. Forsch Komplementarmed Klass Naturheilkd 2004;11(Suppl 1):36–9.

14. Pang PS, Gheorghiade M, Dihu J, et al. Effects of tolvaptan on physician-assessed symptoms and signs in patients hospitalized with acute heart failure syndromes: analysis from the Efficacy of Vasopressin Antagonism in Heart Failure Outcome Study with Tolvaptan (EVEREST) trials. Am Heart J 2011;161:1067–72.

15. Pina IL, Ortiz J. Exercise in heart failure: a review of current applications for testing and training. In: Mann DL, editor. Heart failure: a companion to Braunwald's heart disease. 1st edition. Philadelphia: Saunders; 2004. p. 753–63.

16. LeMaitre JP, Harris S, Hannan J, et al. Maximum oxygen uptake corrected for skeletal muscle mass accurately predicts functional improvements following exercise training in chronic heart failure. Eur J Heart Fail 2006;8:243–8.

17. Davies EJ, Moxham T, Rees K, et al. Exercise based rehabilitation for heart failure. Cochrane Database Syst Rev 2010;(4):CD003331.

18. Bosnak-Guclu M, Arikan H, Savci S, et al. Effects of inspiratory muscle training in patients with heart failure. Respir Med 2011;105:1671–81.

19. Wall HK, Ballard J, Troped P, et al. Impact of home-based, supervised exercise on congestive heart failure. Int J Cardiol 2010;145:267–70.

20. Evans RA, Singh SJ, Collier R, et al. Pulmonary rehabilitation is successful for COPD irrespective of MRC dyspnoea grade. Respir Med 2009;103:1070–5.

21. Pozehl B, Duncan K, Hertzog M. The effects of exercise training on fatigue and dyspnea in heart failure. Eur J Cardiovasc Nurs 2008;7:127–32.

22. Redwine LS, Tsuang M, Rusiewicz A, et al. A pilot study exploring the effects of a 12-week t'ai chi intervention on somatic symptoms of depression in patients with heart failure. J Altern Complement Med 2012;18:744–8.

23. Albert NM, Buchsbaum R, Li J. Randomized study of the effect of video education on heart failure healthcare utilization, symptoms, and self-care behaviors. Patient Educ Couns 2007;69:129–39.

24. Remme WJ, Swedberg K. Guidelines for the diagnosis and treatment of chronic heart failure. Eur Heart J 2001;22:1527–60.

25. Hunt SA, Baker DW, Chin MH, et al. ACC/AHA Guidelines for the evaluation and management of chronic heart failure in the adult: executive summary a report of the American College of Cardiology/American Heart Association Task Force on Practice Guidelines (Committee to Revise the 1995 Guidelines for the Evaluation and Management of Heart Failure): developed in collaboration with the International Society for Heart and Lung Transplantation; Endorsed by the Heart Failure Society of America. Circulation 2001;104:2996–3007.

26. Colin RE, Castillo ML, Orea TA, et al. Effects of a nutritional intervention on body composition, clinical status, and quality of life in patients with heart failure. Nutrition 2004;20:890–5.

27. Naughton MT, Lorenzi-Filho G. Sleep in heart failure. Prog Cardiovasc Dis 2009;51:339–49.

28. Javaheri S. Acetazolamide improves central sleep apnea in heart failure: a double-blind, prospective study. Am J Respir Crit Care Med 2006;173:234–7.

29. Javaheri S, Parker TJ, Wexler L, et al. Effect of theophylline on sleep-disordered breathing in heart failure. N Engl J Med 1996;335:562–7.

30. Andreas S, Clemens C, Sandholzer H, et al. Improvement of exercise capacity with treatment of Cheyne-Stokes respiration in patients with congestive heart failure. J Am Coll Cardiol 1996;27:1486–90.

31. Weiner P, Magadle R, Berar-Yanay N, et al. The cumulative effect of long-acting bronchodilators, exercise, and inspiratory muscle training on the perception of dyspnea in patients with advanced COPD. Chest 2000;118:672–8.

32. Casaburi R, Petty T. Principles and practice of pulmonary rehabilitation. Philadelphia: WB Saunders; 1993.

33. Tashkin DP, Celli B, Senn S, et al. A 4-year trial of tiotropium in chronic obstructive pulmonary disease. N Engl J Med 2008;359:1543–54.

34. Troosters T, Celli B, Lystig T, et al. Tiotropium as a first maintenance drug in COPD: secondary

analysis of the UPLIFT trial. Eur Respir J 2010; 36(1):65–73.

35. O'Donnell DE, Fluge T, Gerken F, et al. Effects of tiotropium on lung hyperinflation, dyspnoea and exercise tolerance in COPD. Eur Respir J 2004; 23:832–40.

36. Niewoehner DE, Rice K, Cote C, et al. Prevention of exacerbations of chronic obstructive pulmonary disease with tiotropium, a once-daily inhaled anticholinergic bronchodilator: a randomized trial. Ann Intern Med 2005;143:317–26.

37. Casaburi R, Kukafka D, Cooper CB, et al. Improvement in exercise tolerance with the combination of tiotropium and pulmonary rehabilitation in patients with COPD. Chest 2005;127:809–17.

38. Casaburi R, Conoscenti CS. Lung function improvements with once-daily tiotropium in chronic obstructive pulmonary disease. Am J Med 2004; 117(Suppl 12A):33S–40S.

39. Casaburi R, Mahler DA, Jones PW, et al. A long-term evaluation of once-daily inhaled tiotropium in chronic obstructive pulmonary disease. Eur Respir J 2002;19:217–24.

40. Sposato B, Franco C. Short term effect of a single dose of formoterol or tiotropium on the isolated nocturnal hypoxemia in stable COPD patients: a double blind randomized study. Eur Rev Med Pharmacol Sci 2008;12:203–11.

41. Aclidinium bromide in chronic obstructive pulmonary disease: NDA 202450. 2012. Available at: http://www.fda.gov/downloads/AdvisoryCommittees/CommitteesMeetingMaterials/Drugs/PulmonaryAllergyDrugsAdvisoryCommittee/UCM294001.pdf. Accessed on April 22, 2013.

42. Alagha K, Bourdin A, Tummino C, et al. An update on the efficacy and safety of aclidinium bromide in patients with COPD. Ther Adv Respir Dis 2011;5:19–28.

43. Mroz RM, Minarowski L, Chyczewska E. Indacaterol add-on therapy improves lung function, exercise capacity and life quality of COPD patients. Adv Exp Med Biol 2013;756:23–8.

44. Spencer SALL, et al. "Health Status Deterioration in Patients with Chronic Obstructive Pulmonary Disease". American Journal of Respiratory and Critical Care Medicine 2001;163(1):122–8.

45. Calverley P, Pauwels R, Vestbo J, et al. Combined salmeterol and fluticasone in the treatment of chronic obstructive pulmonary disease: a randomised controlled trial. Lancet 2003;361:449–56.

46. Calverley PM, Boonsawat W, Cseke Z, et al. Maintenance therapy with budesonide and formoterol in chronic obstructive pulmonary disease. Eur Respir J 2003;22:912–9.

47. Calverley PM, Anderson JA, Celli B, et al. Salmeterol and fluticasone propionate and survival in chronic obstructive pulmonary disease. N Engl J Med 2007;356:775–89.

48. Sharafkhaneh A, Mattewal AS, Abraham VM, et al. Budesonide/formoterol combination in COPD: a US perspective. Int J Chron Obstruct Pulmon Dis 2010;5:357–66.

49. Doherty DE, Tashkin DP, Kerwin E, et al. Effects of mometasone furoate/formoterol fumarate fixed-dose combination formulation on chronic obstructive pulmonary disease (COPD): results from a 52-week phase III trial in subjects with moderate-to-very severe COPD. Int J Chron Obstruct Pulmon Dis 2012;7:57–71.

50. Tashkin DP, Doherty DE, Kerwin E, et al. Efficacy and safety characteristics of mometasone furoate/formoterol fumarate fixed-dose combination in subjects with moderate to very severe COPD: findings from pooled analysis of two randomized, 52-week placebo-controlled trials. Int J Chron Obstruct Pulmon Dis 2012;7:73–86.

51. Spencer MD, Anderson JA. Salmeterol/fluticasone combination produces clinically important benefits in dyspnea and fatigue [abstract]. Am J Respir Crit Care Med 2005;B93.

52. Pulmonary rehabilitation: joint ACCP/AACVPR evidence-based guidelines. ACCP/AACVPR Pulmonary Rehabilitation Guidelines Panel. American College of Chest Physicians. American Association of Cardiovascular and Pulmonary Rehabilitation. Chest 1997;112:1363–96.

53. Lacasse Y, Goldstein R, Lasserson TJ, et al. Pulmonary rehabilitation for chronic obstructive pulmonary disease. Cochrane Database Syst Rev 2006;(4):CD003793.

54. British Thoracic Society Standards of Care Subcommittee on Pulmonary Rehabilitation. Pulmonary rehabilitation. Thorax 2001;56:827–34.

55. Moore J, Fiddler H, Seymour J, et al. Effect of a home exercise video programme in patients with chronic obstructive pulmonary disease. J Rehabil Med 2009;41:195–200.

56. Holland AE, Hill CJ, Conron M, et al. Short term improvement in exercise capacity and symptoms following exercise training in interstitial lung disease. Thorax 2008;63:549–54.

57. Nishiyama O, Kondoh Y, Kimura T, et al. Effects of pulmonary rehabilitation in patients with idiopathic pulmonary fibrosis. Respirology 2008;13:394–9.

58. Weisbord SD, Fried LF, Arnold RM, et al. Prevalence, severity, and importance of physical and emotional symptoms in chronic hemodialysis patients. J Am Soc Nephrol 2005;16:2487–94.

59. Bossola M, Vulpio C, Tazza L. Fatigue in chronic dialysis patients. Semin Dial 2011;24:550–5.

60. McClellan W, Aronoff SL, Bolton WK, et al. The prevalence of anemia in patients with chronic kidney disease. Curr Med Res Opin 2004;20:1501–10.

61. Macdonald JH, Fearn L, Jibani M, et al. Exertional fatigue in patients with CKD. Am J Kidney Dis 2012;60:930–9.

62. Finkelstein FO, Finkelstein SH. Depression in chronic dialysis patients: assessment and treatment. Nephrol Dial Transplant 2000;15:1911–3.

63. Joshwa B, Khakha DC, Mahajan S. Fatigue and depression and sleep problems among hemodialysis patients in a tertiary care center. Saudi J Kidney Dis Transpl 2012;23:729–35.

64. Hedayati SS, Yalamanchili V, Finkelstein FO. A practical approach to the treatment of depression in patients with chronic kidney disease and end-stage renal disease. Kidney Int 2012;81: 247–55.

65. Boulware LE, Liu Y, Fink NE, et al. Temporal relation among depression symptoms, cardiovascular disease events, and mortality in end-stage renal disease: contribution of reverse causality. Clin J Am Soc Nephrol 2006;1:496–504.

66. Merlino G, Piani A, Dolso P, et al. Sleep disorders in patients with end-stage renal disease undergoing dialysis therapy. Nephrol Dial Transplant 2006;21: 184–90.

67. Parker KP, Bliwise DL, Bailey JL, et al. Daytime sleepiness in stable hemodialysis patients. Am J Kidney Dis 2003;41:394–402.

68. Mucsi I, Molnar MZ, Rethelyi J, et al. Sleep disorders and illness intrusiveness in patients on chronic dialysis. Nephrol Dial Transplant 2004;19: 1815–22.

69. Lewis EF, Pfeffer MA, Feng A, et al. Darbepoetin alfa impact on health status in diabetes patients with kidney disease: a randomized trial. Clin J Am Soc Nephrol 2011;6:845–55.

70. Lynch KE, Feldman HI, Berlin JA, et al. Effects of L-carnitine on dialysis-related hypotension and muscle cramps: a meta-analysis. Am J Kidney Dis 2008;52:962–71.

71. Chang Y, Cheng SY, Lin M, et al. The effectiveness of intradialytic leg ergometry exercise for improving sedentary life style and fatigue among patients with chronic kidney disease: a randomized clinical trial. Int J Nurs Stud 2010;47:1383–8.

72. Johansen KL, Painter PL, Sakkas GK, et al. Effects of resistance exercise training and nandrolone decanoate on body composition and muscle function among patients who receive hemodialysis: a randomized, controlled trial. J Am Soc Nephrol 2006;17:2307–14.

73. Chertow GM, Levin NW, Beck GJ, et al. In-center hemodialysis six times per week versus three times per week. N Engl J Med 2010;363: 2287–300.

74. Jaber BL, Lee Y, Collins AJ, et al. Effect of daily hemodialysis on depressive symptoms and post-dialysis recovery time: interim report from the FREEDOM (Following Rehabilitation, Economics and Everyday-Dialysis Outcome Measurements) Study. Am J Kidney Dis 2010;56:531–9.

75. Duarte PS, Miyazaki MC, Blay SL, et al. Cognitive-behavioral group therapy is an effective treatment for major depression in hemodialysis patients. Kidney Int 2009;76:414–21.

76. Horigan A, Rocchiccioli J, Trimm D. Dialysis and fatigue: implications for nurses–a case study analysis. Medsurg Nurs 2012;21:158–63, 175.

77. Swain MG. Fatigue in liver disease: pathophysiology and clinical management. Can J Gastroenterol 2006;20:181–8.

78. Kumar D, Tandon RK. Fatigue in cholestatic liver disease–a perplexing symptom. Postgrad Med J 2002;78:404–7.

79. Huet PM, Deslauriers J, Tran A, et al. Impact of fatigue on the quality of life of patients with primary biliary cirrhosis. Am J Gastroenterol 2000; 95:760–7.

80. Newton JL. Fatigue in primary biliary cirrhosis. Clin Liver Dis 2008;12:367–83.

81. Anderson K, Jones DE, Wilton K, et al. Restless leg syndrome is a treatable cause of sleep disturbance and fatigue in primary biliary cirrhosis. Liver Int 2013;33:239–43.

82. Poynard T, Cacoub P, Ratziu V, et al. Fatigue in patients with chronic hepatitis C. J Viral Hepat 2002;9: 295–303.

83. Newton JL. Systemic symptoms in non-alcoholic fatty liver disease. Dig Dis 2010;28:214–9.

84. Kalaitzakis E, Josefsson A, Castedal M, et al. Factors related to fatigue in patients with cirrhosis before and after liver transplantation. Clin Gastroenterol Hepatol 2012;10:174–81, 181.e1.

85. Montagnese S, Nsemi LM, Cazzagon N, et al. Sleep-wake profiles in patients with primary biliary cirrhosis. Liver Int 2013;33:203–9.

86. Sarkar S, Jiang Z, Evon DM, et al. Fatigue before, during and after antiviral therapy of chronic hepatitis C: results from the Virahep-C study. J Hepatol 2012;57:946–52.

87. Nishino S, Mignot E. Wake-promoting medications: basic mechanism and pharmacology. In: Kryger MH, Roth T, Dement WC, editors. Principles and practice of sleep medicine. St Louis (MO): Elsevier Saunders; 2011. p. 510–26.

88. O'Malley MB, Gleeson SK, Weir ID. Wake-promoting medications: efficacy and adverse effects. In: Kryger MH, Roth T, Dement WC, editors. Principles and practice of sleep medicine. St Louis (MO): Elsevier Saunders; 2011. p. 527–41.

89. Koob GF, Sanna PP, Bloom FE. Neuroscience of addiction. Neuron 1998;21:467–76.

90. Koob GF. Drugs of abuse: anatomy, pharmacology and function of reward pathways. Trends Pharmacol Sci 1992;13:177–84.

91. Davis JM, Kopin IJ, Lemberger L, et al. Effects of urinary pH on amphetamine metabolism. Ann N Y Acad Sci 1971;179:493–501.

92. Faraj BA, Israili ZH, Perel JM, et al. Metabolism and disposition of methylphenidate-14C: studies in man and animals. J Pharmacol Exp Ther 1974; 191:535–47.

93. Guilleminault C. Amphetamines and narcolepsy: use of the Stanford database. Sleep 1993;16: 199–201.

94. Vignatelli L, D'Alessandro R, Candelise L. Antidepressant drugs for narcolepsy. Cochrane Database Syst Rev 2008;(1):CD003724.

95. Guilleminault C, Mancuso J, Salva MA, et al. Viloxazine hydrochloride in narcolepsy: a preliminary report. Sleep 1986;9:275–9.

96. Lin JS, Roussel B, Akaoka H, et al. Role of catecholamines in modafinil and amphetamine induced wakefulness, a comparative pharmacological study. Brain Res 1992;591:2319–26.

97. Mignot E, Nishino S, Guilleminault C, et al. Modafinil binds to the dopamine uptake carrier site with low affinity. Sleep 1994;17:436–7.

98. Ferraro L, Tanganelli S, O'Connor WT, et al. The vigilance promoting drug modafinil increases dopamine release in the rat nucleus accumbens via the involvement of a local GABAergic mechanism. Eur J Pharmacol 1996;306:33–9.

99. Ishizuka T, Murakami M, Yamatodani A. Involvement of central histaminergic systems in modafinil-induced but not methylphenidate-induced increases in locomotor activity in rats. Eur J Pharmacol 2008;578:209–15.

100. Ishizuka T, Sakamoto Y, Sakurai T, et al. Modafinil increases histamine release in the anterior hypothalamus of rats. Neurosci Lett 2003;339: 143–6.

101. Mendelson W. Hypnotic medications: mechanisms of action and pharmacologic effects. In: Kryger MH, Roth T, Dement WC, editors. Principles and practice of sleep medicine. St Louis (MO): Elsevier Saunders; 2011. p. 483–91.

102. Hirshkowitz M, Rose MW, Sharafkhaneh A. Neurotransmitters, neurochemistry, and the clinical pharmacology of sleep. In: Chokroverty S, editor. Sleep disorders medicine. 3rd edition. Philadelphia: Saunders Elsevier; 2009. p. 67–79.

103. Foster S, Johnson RL. Desk reference to nature's medicine. Washington, DC: National Geographic; 2006.

Index

Note: Page numbers of article titles are in **boldface** type.

sleep.theclinics.com

Printed and bound by CPI Group (UK) Ltd, Croydon, CR0 4YY

03/10/2024

01040354-0002